Table of Contents

For *Adult Fitness Examination: A Physical Therapy Approach*

Physical activity is a powerful intervention, as evidenced by the plethora of studies indicating its relationship to morbidity and mortality in both well populations and populations with functional limitations, impairments, or disabilities. More important, physically active adults report greater quality of life and enhanced productivity in vocational and leisure pursuits. As experts in prescribing and applying physical activity interventions, physical therapists are well positioned to increase the physical fitness of adults—the state that results from regular physical activity or inactivity. To that end, physical therapist and educator Dan Millrood, PT, EdM, has written the first physical therapy-specific workbook providing the tools physical therapists can use to assess adult physical fitness.

Federal and local governments, employers, insurers, health systems, and providers are being called on to better manage the state of "dis-ease" of the American public, and this workbook will be a welcome addition to the tool box of physical therapists who have a very important role to play to achieve the goal of improving the physical fitness of the adult public. While the Adult Fitness Examination is targeted for healthy adults, it's a starting point for tools that examine different populations. I applaud Dan Millrood for his foresight and contribution to this physical activity imperative.

—Janet Bezner, PT, DPT, PhD
Vice President, Education, and Vice President, Governance and Administration, APTA
Former Program Director, Doctor of Science Program in Health Promotion and Wellness,
Rocky Mountain University of Health Professions, Provo, Utah
Former Vice President, PeakCare Inc, a wellness technology consulting firm

Impressive! *Adult Fitness Examination: A Physical Therapy Approach* comes at a critical juncture in our profession. It would be difficult to identify a profession more prepared and effectively able to meet the growing needs of our society in reference to personal health and wellness than physical therapists. We have the background, the credibility, and the relationships. And now, thanks to this new book, we have a valuable tool in helping us address those needs. The Adult Fitness Examination doesn't just introduce the concept and stop there. Instead, it provides the tools and resources to almost immediately jump in and get started in the *right* way. Within the cover of this book, physical therapists have everything necessary to move forward in establishing a baseline of health and wellness for their clients. If you're serious about getting started in providing a comprehensive fitness evaluation as part of your practice, this is a must resource.

—Brad Cooper, PT, MSPT, MBA, MTC, ATC, CWC
CEO, Wellness Coach Catalyst (www.WellnessCoachCatalyst.com)
Author, Employee Wellness: Implementing a High Impact, High ROI Strategy

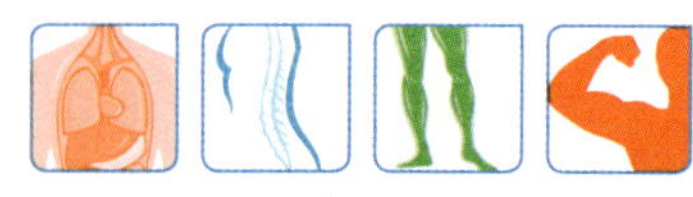

About the Authors:

Daniel Millrood, PT, EdM, has been practicing, teaching, and promoting physical therapist practice and research that focuses on preventive health care, injury prevention, health promotion, physical fitness, and wellness for the last 3 decades. After receiving an undergraduate degree in biopsychology from Columbia College in 1986 and a master's degree in physical therapy from Columbia College of Physicians and Surgeons in 1988, Millrood received a master's degree in applied physiology from Columbia University's Teachers College under the advisement of Ronald Demeersman, PhD, and Jason Mateika, PhD. He continues his doctoral work at Teachers College in applied physiology. During his high school and collegiate tenure, Millrood also held several state and regional powerlifting titles and was ranked nationally.

Millrood's interest and passion for physical therapy in preventive health care and wellness evolved while practicing in a variety of settings where many patients and clients were treated for injury and disease that resulted from of a lack of physical fitness and general conditioning. This served as the inspiration for the Adult Fitness Examination, which Millrood started developing in the early 1990s.

Millrood created, implemented, and directed the academic and research coursework for physical therapy in preventive health care and wellness for the Doctor of Physical Therapy Program at New York Medical College in 2005. Millrood also brought his coursework to the DPT and t-DPT programs at Dominican College in New York, where he currently teaches. Millrood continues to provide educational coursework for clinical implementation of physical therapy in preventive health care and wellness for postprofessional continuing education coursework.

Millrood currently owns an outpatient private practice that emphasizes physical therapy as an integral component of a multidisciplinary health care team that focuses on obesity and diabetes prevention and treatment, in addition to general community-based health promotion, injury prevention, and wellness interventions across the lifespan. He also has an avid interest in health care consumer advocacy, and owns and operates an organic farm that promotes healthy living through community-supported agricultural programs. It is Millrood's hope and dream that physical therapist practice will continue to evolve to promote public health through preventive services in addition to the rehabilitative services that physical therapists typically provide.

Charlotte Chua, PT, DPT, is the director of physical therapy at Queens Boulevard Extended Care Facility in Woodside, NY. Chua completed her doctoral thesis at New York Medical College under the advisement of Daniel Millrood, PT, EdM, and graduated summa cum laude in 2005 as a member of the college's first-ever DPT class. Chua's thesis provided foundational work for the Adult Fitness Examination. Chua is recognized as a master clinician by New York University, serving as a clinical instructor for students throughout the Northeast.

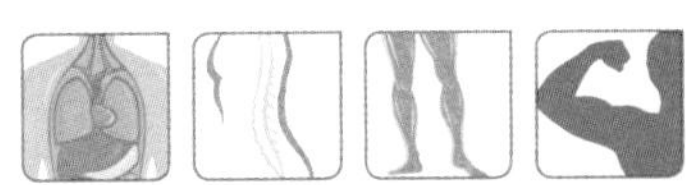

Authors' Acknowledgments:

I would like to thank my father, Bernard Millrood, MD, a general practitioner of family medicine, for teaching me to provide care for those in need and that all health ailments cannot be cured by pills, needles, or knives. I would also like to thank my entire family, including my extended family of colleagues and friends who have been chronically exposed to discourse on the role of physical therapy in preventive health care, wellness, and public health. I would l to give an extra-special thanks to Lori Zalner, PT, Michael Majsak, PT, EdD, Kathleen Edinger, PT, Christina Rosado, PT, Julie Fineman PT, EdM, as well as my co-author Charlotte Chua, PT, DPT, for all of the encouragement, support, and feedback throughout the development of the Adult Fitness Examination. I would also like to thank the countless students, field clinicians, and content experts who have provided valuable input during this process. Special thanks a also due to Karen Segal, PhD, Ronald Demeersman, PhD, and Jason Mateika, PhD, for nurturing, inspiring, and infec me with a love and passion for applied physiology. Most important, love and thanks go to my wonderful wife Crimora and my sons Isaac and Lucas for sacrificing precious hours for a good cause. And the greatest thanks to Janet Bezn PT, PhD, vice president, education, governance, and administration, Lois Douthitt, senior director of publishing and member communications, and everyone at the American Physical Therapy Association for dedicating their service ar time to promoting the evolution of the role of physical therapy in the preventive health care arena and for encouragi me to publish this work.

—Dan Millrood, PT, [illegible]

I would like to extend my sincerest love and thanks to the following people for all their support: to my parents and family for making me who I am; to Dan Millrood for always thinking outside of the box; to my professors at New York Medical College and my clinical instructors for helping me develop my skills as a clinician; to my fellow classmates fo all of their emotional support and guidance; and to Jeff for always being by my side forever.

—Charlotte Chua, PT, [illegible]

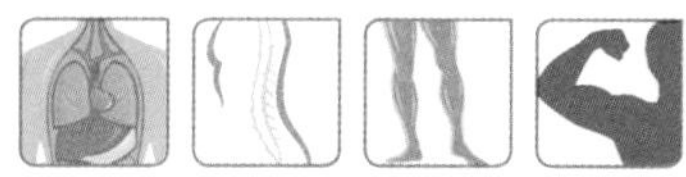

Foreword

It is almost incomprehensible that despite ongoing advances in biomedical, pharmaceutical, and information systems technologies, the current health care system in the United States of America is failing. The United States spends more per capita on health care than any other nation. The incidence and/or cost of managing obesity, heart disease, type 2 diabetes mellitus, osteoarthritis (OA), and cancer are enormous. The statistics are staggering:

- According to the American Heart Association, the direct and indirect costs of medical treatment related to heart disease (suffered by 1 in 3 Americans), was $444 billion in 2010.[1]

- The Centers for Disease Control and Prevention reported in 2009 that chronic disease accounts for about 75% of the nation's aggregate health care spending—or $5,300 per person each year. In taxpayer-funded programs, treatment of chronic disease constitutes an even larger proportion of spending—96 cents per dollar for Medicare and 83 cents per dollar for Medicaid.[2]

- The journal *Arthritis and Rheumatism* reported that in 2009 the cost of health care related to OA was $185.5 billion.[3]

- A 2011 study by the Society of Actuaries estimates the United States spends $270 billion per year in preventable health care costs, lost productivity, disability, and premature death from chronic conditions related to overweight and obesity.

Meanwhile, consumers have little confidence in the current health care system. Something must be done. The Patient Protection and Affordable Care Act of 2011 may or may not have been the answer, but the triple aims of health care reform—focusing on cost, access, and quality of care—are solid. A system that emphasizes preventive, patient-centered care, provided and managed by a multidisciplinary team of providers that includes physical therapists (PTs) as specialists on movement and function, is a solution that would allow our health care system to cost-effectively maximize the amazing resources we have at our fingertips.

APTA envisions physical therapists as primary-point practitioners in the preventive health care arena. To achieve that vision, PTs must be aggressively trained at entry level and postprofessionally. How can physical therapist educators, clinicians, and researchers approach this task?

When I started practicing physical therapy in the late 1980s, referrals for our services were typically generated by other health care team members, after disease or injury already had affected patients and their families, caregivers, and third-party payers. It was clear to me that skilled physical therapist services prior to the onset of injury, disease, and illness, including direct intervention and patient education, could have helped prevent the unwanted suffering and loss of quality of life that resulted from a lack of physical fitness. There was, however, no industry standard, no formal training, no physical therapy-based approach to address this need. This realization led to the development of a physical therapy-based adult fitness examination, a tool that can assess fitness parameters that are related to injury, disease, a lack of wellness, decreased function, and a reduction in quality of life. The foundational thought process was that PTs could identify and address factors that frequently contribute to injury, disease, and the increased cost of care related to treating preventable conditions.

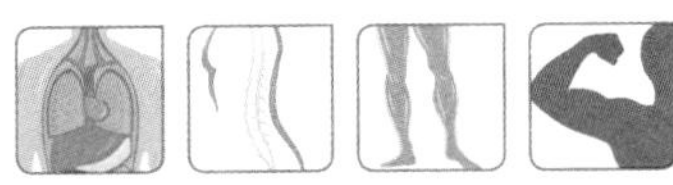

The ongoing rise of the clinical doctorate, direct access, and autonomous physical therapist practice brings great opportunity to our profession. The recent evolution of health care as a commodity enables PTs to meet the market demand for a less invasive, more cost-effective product that produces better outcomes. By using fitness assessment tools across the lifespan, PTs can obtain baseline and follow-up measurements of specific fitness parameters related to public health; these can educate and train patients and clients in individually tailored exercise programs that address potential fitness impairments that can result in costly injury and disease. The provision of evidence-based care, with related measureable outcomes, could allow PTs to have a great impact in the future of health care.

As PTs seize this promising opportunity offered during the rapid evolution of the American health care system, we can cement an important role on the multidisciplinary health care team into the future, ensuring our participation in an effective approach to improved health for our patients and clients at a reduced cost and, thus, the employment of physical therapy clinicians, during a transition that will bring deep cuts in unnecessary services and related costs.

It is the dawn of a new era that will allow physical therapy to flourish and provide maximal impact on the health care system. We have studied and trained hard. It is time for us to embrace this opportunity. Please enjoy this text as it guides you through a new way of thinking and a new method of examination that will allow physical therapist clinicians the chance to offer our patients and clients everything we can offer to help—person-by-person rather than body part-by-body part. By examining and treating the whole patient in a comprehensive, cost-effective, evidence-based approach that uses measurable outcomes, we can maximize the impact we can have on the lives of our patients and clients.

REFERENCES

1. American Heart Association. *Forecasting the Future of Cardiovascular Disease in the United States.* A Policy Statement From the American Heart Association; 2011. http://circ.ahajournals.org/content/123/8/933.full. Accessed July 23, 2012.
2. Centers for Disease Control and Prevention. Chronic Diseases: The Power to Prevent, The Call to Control: At a Glance 2009. Webpage. http://www.cdc.gov/chronicdisease/resources/publications/AAG/chronic.htm. Accessed July 23, 2012.
3. Kotlarz H, Gunnarsson CL, Fang H, Rizzo JA. Insurer and Out-of-Pocket Costs of Osteoarthritis in the US: Evidence From National Survey Data. *Arthritis and Rheumatism.* 2009;60(12):3546-3553.

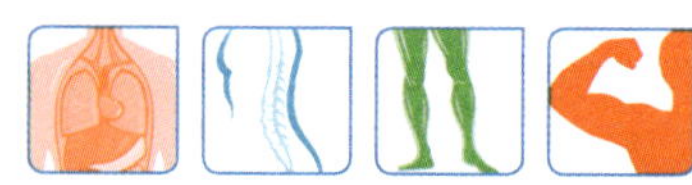

Adult Fitness Examination: A Physical Therapy Approach

The Adult Fitness Examination (AFE) contained in *Adult Fitness Examination: A Physical Therapy Approach* is a comprehensive, noninvasive, evidence-based physical therapy approach to assessing the fitness of asymptomatic adults. It incorporates fitness components of musculoskeletal alignment, balance, range of motion, and manual muscle testing that are not addressed by the American College of Sports Medicine (ACSM). The AFE measures functional performance and uses common physical therapy tests and measures. The AFE can be used to monitor wellness outcomes over time and promotes interdisciplinary communication regarding adult fitness.

Adult Fitness Examination: A Physical Therapy Approach comprises the following sections:

- **General Overview**—The background information about the structure and components of the AFE.
- **Instructions**—Step-by-step directions on how to conduct the tests and measures, as well as normative data.
- **Workbook**—The physical therapist uses it during the test to document findings of the AFE.
- **Client Take-Home Form**—An easy-to-understand guide about the AFE and the results of the evaluation. The therapist fills it out and gives to the patient/client with recommended activities and exercises to address areas of weakness while maintaining/improving all other areas.

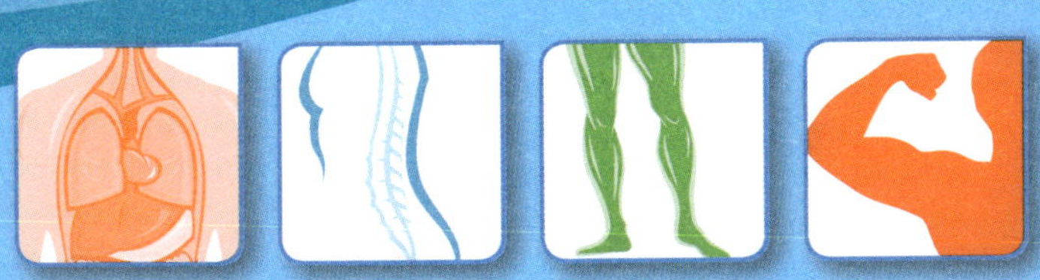

General Overview of the Adult Fitness Examination

Physical therapists (PTs) are health care providers that play an increasingly important role in health promotion, injury prevention, and wellness. APTA's *Guide to Physical Therapist Practice*, 2nd edition, states that physical therapists "provide prevention and promote health, wellness, and fitness."[1(p32)] APTA's Vision 2020 states that physical therapists should emerge as practitioners of choice for health promotion, injury prevention, fitness, and wellness.[2] A growing number of physical therapists are voicing interest and actively practicing to promote health and prevent injury across the client's lifespan. Simultaneously, academicians are developing curricula that will prepare physical therapist students and post-professionals to be practitioners of choice for prevention of impairments in body functions and structures, activity limitations, and participation restrictions (collectively termed "disability").

The academic and clinical training that prepares PTs to serve a key role in preventive health care and wellness provides many evaluative tools and techniques that PTs can use to assess adult fitness. Traditionally, physical therapy services are sought when a person has difficulty with daily functional activities, and PTs gauge how an individual deviates from the general population. PTs can use these same skills and methods to determine an asymptomatic individual's current level of physical fitness as well as gauge changes in the individual over time. A standardized, physical therapy-based fitness examination tool to determine the overall physical fitness level of an adult client can provide clinicians with data that can be used to educate and guide clients to better health, while facilitating a continuum of care within a multidisciplinary, team-based health care model.

PTs, other health care providers, and third-party payers can share standardized and universally accepted client fitness measures to optimize physical wellness outcomes. In addition, gearing treatment toward early intervention and prevention has the potential to reduce overall health care costs by monitoring a client's fitness level and addressing potential problems. The Adult Fitness Examination (AFE) contained herein was developed in response to this need. The AFE synthesizes evidence-based, entry-level PT examination techniques and measures into a cost-effective, user-friendly, clinically relevant protocol that can be administered to an adult wellness client.

The AFE was developed to determine physical fitness levels for asymptomatic individuals 18–65 years of age, using common physical therapy tests and measures to quantify and qualify key components of physical health and wellness. Significant components of physical health and wellness are[3]:

- Cardiovascular/Cardiorespiratory Fitness
- Musculoskeletal Alignment and Development
- Body Composition
- Musculoskeletal Fitness
- Muscular Strength and Endurance
- Balance
- Aerobic Endurance

The AFE is designed to be conducted by a PT in a typical clinical setting. The tests and measures are structured for efficiency and safety, beginning with a preparticipation screening.

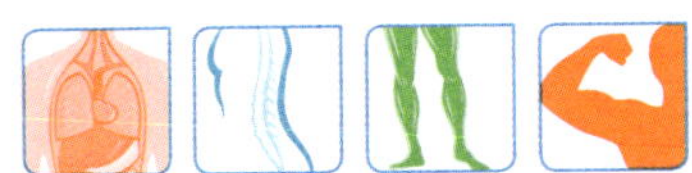

PREPARTICIPATION HEALTH SCREENING AND CLIENT INFORMATION

The client completes the Physical Activity Readiness Questionnaire (PAR-Q)[4] and the ACSM Health/Fitness Facility preparticipation screening questionnaire[5,6] to ensure client safety and appropriateness for exercise testing, and to screen for the need to refer the client to a physician. If the client is safe to continue, the PT obtains client information such as current health status, exercise habits, and medical history.

CARDIOVASCULAR/CARDIORESPIRATORY FITNESS (PART I)

Cardio-vagal tone is an important aspect of cardiovascular/cardiorespiratory fitness. Stimulation of the vagus nerve, which carries approximately 80% of all parasympathetic fibers, induces relaxation of vasculature and myocardial tissue.[7] Maintenance of optimal vagal tone reduces the risk of cardiovascular disease.

- **Resting Heart Rate**—This is a common measure of cardio-vagal tone. The PT assesses baseline measures of heart rate.
- **Resting Blood Pressure**—This is a common measure of cardio-vagal tone. The PT assesses baseline measures of blood pressure.

MUSCULOSKELETAL ALIGNMENT AND DEVELOPMENT

Musculoskeletal alignment and development are important to an individual's overall health in that misalignment can lead to pain; can adversely affect balance, gait, strength, and function; and can lead to degenerative joint changes. Ideally, proper musculoskeletal alignment is the state in which a person's joints experience minimal stress while at rest, with minimal muscle activity required to maintain the at-rest position.

- **Visual Inspection of Posture With Plumb Line**—The PT observes the client's alignment and muscle development using a plumb line from different views.

BODY COMPOSITION

It is well documented and highly publicized that obesity is a major health issue and increases the risk for morbidities such as hypertension, diabetes mellitus, stroke, and coronary artery disease. Direct measures of body composition typically are not performed in physical therapy clinics due to the high costs of equipment and certification. However, anthropometric measures such as body mass index (BMI) and waist circumference (WC) are easily obtainable. Because there are standard classifications for these measures, their values can be used to determine levels of risk of morbidity and mortality for the client.

- **Body Mass Index With Waist Circumference**—The relationship of these 2 measurements is stratified into disease risk categories developed by the National Institutes of Health and the National Heart, Lung and Blood Institute.[8,9] The PT uses a scale and tape measure to obtain measurements.

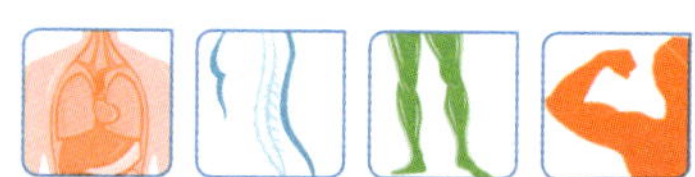

MUSCULOSKELETAL FITNESS

Musculoskeletal fitness comprises 3 elements: flexibility, strength, and endurance. Flexibility is the ability to move through a range of motion (ROM) without restriction from soft tissue, or capsular or connective tissue elements.[5] Strength is the ability of the muscle to generate maximal force and carry out work against a force.[5,10] Endurance is the ability of a muscle to perform repeated contractions over time until fatigue.[5] Poor muscle flexibility is associated with possible risk of injury and joint disease/pathology. Poor muscle strength can contribute to possible injury.

Muscular Flexibility

- **Gross Range-of-Motion (ROM) Screen**—The PT conducts a general overview of the client's joint mobility and flexibility to gain a quick impression of the client's overall flexibility and to highlight any deviations.
- **Apley's Scratch Test**—This test further investigates the client's ROM in a functional manner. The test combines shoulder flexion, internal rotation with adduction of 1 arm, and shoulder extension, external rotation with abduction of the other arm.[11] These motions are used daily for activities including fastening a bra or reaching for a wallet in a back pocket.
- **YMCA Sit-and-Reach Test**—This test assesses overall lower body flexibility. The PT performs it in lieu of other sit-and-reach tests that require specific equipment not always available in physical therapy clinics.

Muscular Strength and Endurance

- **Gross Manual Muscle Tests**—The PT conducts this test to gain a general impression of the client's overall strength and to highlight any deviations.
- **Handgrip Strength**—This measure has been linked to general upper body strength and the prediction of disability and mortality.[12] The PT gauges handgrip strength using a hand dynamometer.
- **Curl-Up Test**—This test commonly is used to evaluate abdominal strength and endurance.
- **Push-Up Test**—This test commonly is used to evaluate gross upper-body strength and endurance.
- **Unilateral Step-Down Test**—The PT conducts this test as a functional weight-bearing activity to assess strength and endurance of the lower body and lower extremities.

BALANCE

Balance is a major fitness component commonly overlooked during routine physical examination. It is integral to everyday function, as gravity is a constant force. Maintaining balance in the upright position requires complex integration of various systems—the vestibular, somatosensory, and visual systems. Balance is required for activities of daily living, such as those that include lifting or bending. Impaired balance contributes to falls, which can lead to impairments and possible disability. Walking can be thought of as controlled falling. Eighty percent of the gait cycle is spent on a single limb.[13,14] The activity of walking is not always on a smooth surface or in a linear pattern, and at times a person's stride length changes to accommodate the environment, such as walking from rock to rock across a stream or avoiding a pothole in the middle of the sidewalk.

- **Single Limb Stance Test**—The PT conducts this test with the client's eyes open and closed to assess the vestibular, somatosensory, and visual systems.
- **Upper Extremity Functional Reach Test**—Reaching for objects is a common daily activity. The Upper Extremity Reach Test has been linked to prediction of future falls.[15]
- **Lower Extremity Functional Reach Test**—This test assesses the client's ability to reach with 1 leg as far as possible in several directions while maintaining balance on the other leg.

CARDIOVASCULAR/CARDIORESPIRATORY FITNESS (PART II)

Sustained physical activity requires energy for the muscles to function, and that energy comes from oxygen. As the degree of work increases, so does the need to supply oxygen to the functioning muscles. The condition of the cardiovascular/cardiorespiratory systems will dictate the efficacy of energy delivery and, thus, the performance of the task. Poor cardiovascular/respiratory fitness can result in cardiovascular disease, decreased function, and increased morbidity/mortality.

- **Submaximal Bruce Protocol for Predicted VO2max**—One method of assessing cardiovascular/cardiorespiratory fitness is maximal aerobic power or maximal oxygen consumption (VO2max), the maximum amount of oxygen the body can consume at the highest exercise intensity. A higher VO2max is desired indicating the efficacy of the cardiovascular/cardiorespiratory system in delivering oxygen to working muscles. The commonly performed test for determination of VO2max is a maximal effort treadmill test with gas analyzer and an echocardiogram (ECG),[5,7,16] but it is not feasible to safely conduct the test in a typical physical therapy setting. Since heart rate at any given workload can be correlated with O2 uptake, the PT can extrapolate a predicted VO2 value resulting from a submaximal test. The primary advantage of a submaximal VO2 test is less effort by the patient/client, meaning less risk of injury or medical conditions that can result from exhaustion. The PT conducts the submaximal Bruce Protocol test using a treadmill.[17,18]
- **Heart Rate Recovery**—In addition to resting vitals, heart rate recovery (HRR) activity is also an important measure of cardio-vagal tone, since it measures how rapidly the heart rate declines over a period of time from an excited state. In healthy trained individuals post-exercise, the heart rate will decrease at a faster rate than normal because cardio-vagal function is more efficient, resulting in a greater parasympathetic effect on the body. In the Framingham Heart Study, a rapid HRR after exercise was associated with lower risk of CHD and CVD.[19] A slower heart rate recovery indicates decreased cardio-vagal activity, which is a risk factor for death.[20-23]

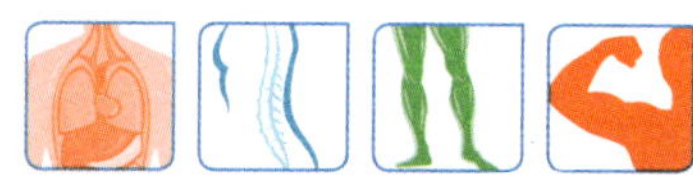

REFERENCES

1. Guide to physical therapist practice, second edition. *Phys Ther.* 2001;81:9-744.
2. American Physical Therapy Association. APTA Vision Statement for Physical Therapy 2020 (HOD P06-00-24-35). Alexandria, VA: American Physical Therapy Association; 2000. http://www.apta.org/AM/Template.cfm?Section=Home&TEMPLATE=/CM/HTMLDisplay.cfm&CONTENTID=33814. Accessed July 7, 2009.
3. President's Council on Physical Fitness. Definitions: Health, Fitness, and Physical Activity. PCPFS Research Digests. Washington, DC: President's Council on Physical Fitness; 2000. http://www.fitness.gov/digest_mar2000.htm. Accessed December 3, 2010.
4. Physical Activity Readiness Questionnaire (PAR-Q) and You. Canadian Society for Exercise Physiology website. http://www.csep.ca/CMFiles/publications/parq/par-q.pdf. Accessed May 19, 2010.
5. American College of Sports Medicine. *ACSM's Guidelines for Exercise Testing and Prescription.* 8th ed. Philadelphia, PA: Lippincott Williams & Wilkins; 2010.
6. American College of Sports Medicine. *ACSM's Health-Related Physical Fitness Assessment Manual.* 7th ed. Baltimore, MD: Lippincott Williams & Wilkins; 2006.
7. McArdleWD, Katch FI, Katch VL. *Exercise Physiology.* 5th ed. Baltimore, MD: Lippincott Williams & Wilkins; 2001.
8. National Heart, Lung and Blood Institute. *JNC VII Express: The Seventh Report of the Joint National Committee on Prevention, Detection, Evaluation, and Treatment of High Blood Pressure.* Washington, DC: National Institutes of Health, US Department of Health and Human Services; 2003. http://www.nhlbi.nih.gov/guidelines/hypertension/express.pdf. Accessed August 25, 2009.
9. National Heart, Lung and Blood Institute. *Clinical Guidelines on the Identification, Evaluation, and Treatment of Overweight and Obesity in Adults: Body Mass Index Table.* Washington, DC: National Institutes of Health, US Department of Health and Human Services; 1998. http://www.nhlbi.nih.gov/guidelines/obesity/bmi_tbl.htm Accessed August 25, 2009.
10. Kisner C, Colby LA. *Therapeutic Exercise: Foundations and Techniques.* 4th ed. Philadelphia, PA: F A Davis Co; 2002.
11. Magee DJ. *Orthopedic Physical Assessment.* 4th ed. Philadelphia, PA: Saunders; 2002.
12. Payne N, Gledhill N, Katzmarzyk PT, Jamnik V, Ferguson S. Health implications of musculoskeletal fitness. *Can J Appl Physiol.* 2000;25(2):114-126.
13. Ranchos Los Amigos. *Gait: Observational Gait Analysis.* Downey, CA: Los Amigos Research and Education Inc; 2000.
14. Sudarsky L. Geriatrics: gait disorders in the elderly. *N Eng J Med.* 1990;322(20):1441-1446.
15. Duncan PW, Studenski S, Chandler J, Prescott B. Functional reach: predictive validity in a sample of elderly male veterans. *J Gerontol.* 1992;47(3):M93-M98.
16. Pollock ML, Wilmore JH. *Exercise in Health and Disease: Evaluation and Prescription for Prevention and Rehabilitation.* 2nd ed. Philadelphia, PA: WB Saunders Co; 1990.
17. Vehrs PR, George JD, Fellingham GW, Plowman SA, Dustman-Allen K. Submaximal treadmill exercise test to predict VO2max in fit adults. *Meas Phys Ed Exerc Sci.* 2007;11:2,61-72.
18. Bruce RA, Kusumi F, Hosmer D. Maximal oxygen intake and nomographic assessment of functional aerobic impairment in cardiovascular disease. *Am Heart J.* 1973;85:546–562.
19. Morshedi-Meibodi A, Larson MG, Levy D, O'Donnell CJ, Vasan RS. Heart rate recovery after treadmill exercise testing and risk of cardiovascular disease events (the Framingham heart study). *Am J Cardiol.* 2002;90(8):848-852.
20. Aktas MK, Ozduran V, Pothier CE, Lang R, Lauer MS. Global risk scores and exercise testing for predicting all-cause mortality in a preventive medicine program. *JAMA.* 2004;292(12):1462-1468.
21. Cole CR, Blackstone EH, Pashkow FJ, Snader CE, Lauer MS. Heart-rate recovery immediately after exercise as a predictor of mortality. *N Eng J Med.* 1999;341:1351-1357.
22. Desai MY, De La Pena-Almaguer E, Mannting F. Abnormal heart rate recovery after exercise: a comparison with known indicators of increased mortality. *Cardiol.* 2001;96(1):38-44.
23. Mora S, Redberg RF, Cui Y, et al. Ability of exercise testing to predict cardiovascular and all-cause death in asymptomatic women: a 20-year follow-up of the lipid research clinics prevalence study. *JAMA.* 2003;290(12):1600-1607.

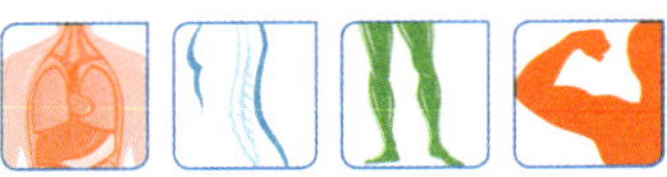

Components of the Adult Fitness Examination

Component	Tests
CARDIOVASCULAR/ CARDIORESPIRATORY FITNESS (PART I)	▪ Resting Heart Rate ▪ Resting Blood Pressure
MUSCULOSKELETAL ALIGNMENT AND DEVELOPMENT	▪ Visual Inspection of Posture With Plumb Line
BODY COMPOSITION	▪ Body Mass Index ▪ Waist Circumference
MUSCULOSKELETAL FITNESS: MUSCULAR FLEXIBILITY	▪ UE/LE Range-of-Motion Screen ▪ Apley's Scratch Test ▪ YMCA Sit-and-Reach Test
MUSCULOSKELETAL FITNESS: MUSCULAR STRENGTH AND ENDURANCE	▪ UE/LE Muscle Strength Tests ▪ Handgrip Strength ▪ Curl-Up Test ▪ Push-Up Test ▪ Unilateral Step-Down Test
BALANCE	▪ Single Limb Stance Test ▪ UE Functional Reach Test ▪ LE Functional Reach Test
CARDIOVASCULAR/ CARDIORESPIRATORY FITNESS (PART II)	▪ Submaximal Bruce Protocol for Predicted VO2max and Heart Rate Recovery

Equipment/Supply Checklist

- ☐ Exam table
- ☐ Floor mats
- ☐ Hand dynamometer
- ☐ Heart rate monitor (optional)
- ☐ Masking tape
- ☐ Metronome
- ☐ Plumb line (string, weight, attachment)
- ☐ Sphygmomanometer
- ☐ Screening questionnaires
- ☐ Step stool
- ☐ Stethoscope
- ☐ Stopwatch
- ☐ Tape measure
- ☐ Treadmill
- ☐ Weight scale
- ☐ Yardstick or ruler

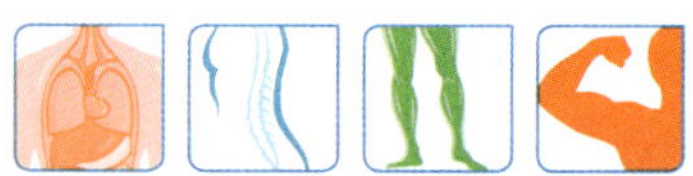

Adult Fitness Examination: Instructions

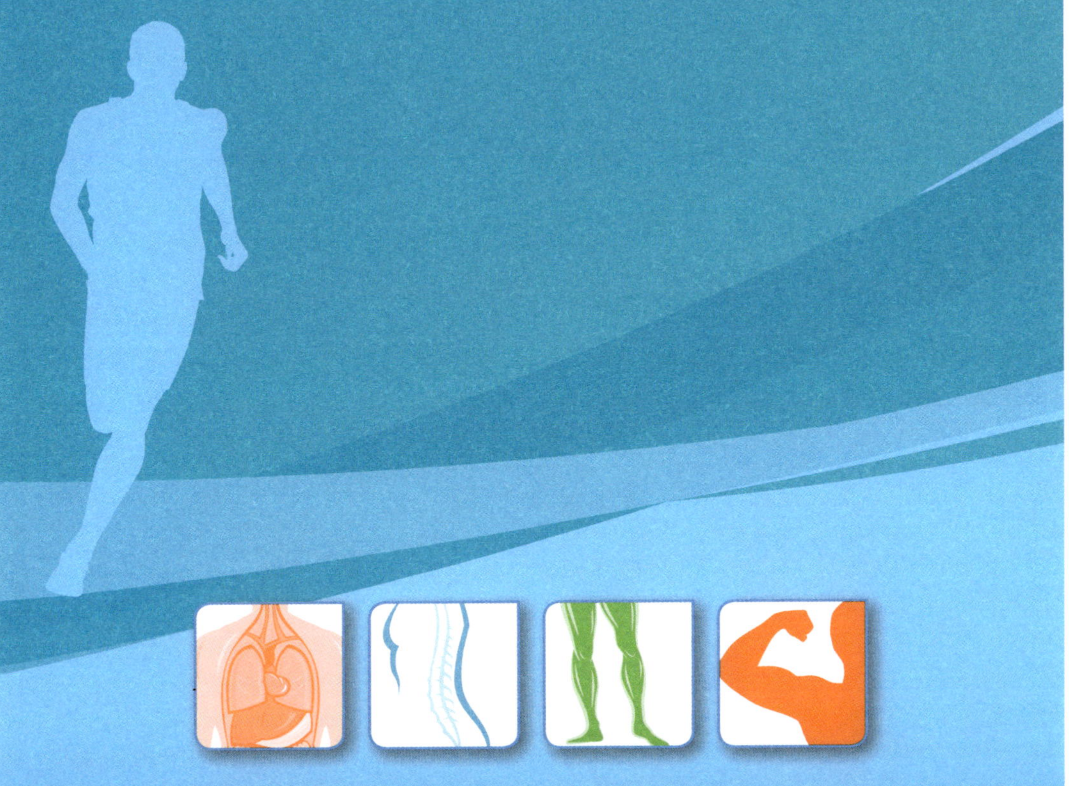

Preparticipation Health Screening and Client Information

ITEMS NEEDED: PHYSICAL ACTIVITY READINESS QUESTIONNAIRE (PAR-Q), AHA/ACSM HEALTH/FITNESS FACILITY PREPARTICIPATION SCREENING QUESTIONNAIRE

1. Instruct client to fill out the **Physical Activity Readiness Questionnaire (PAR-Q) on page 31 of the workbook** and the American Health Association/American College of Sports Medicine (AHA/ACSM) **Health/Fitness Facility Preparticipation Screening Questionnaire on page 32 of the workbook** prior to client interview.

2. If client is cleared for exercise participation according to the criteria of the PAR-Q and AHA/ACSM and/or by physician's medical clearance, initiate the Adult Fitness Examination (AFE).

3. **Document the following information using the worksheet on page 33:**
   - Client's name and sex
   - Date the AFE is being conducted
   - Client's hand dominance
   - Client's age
   - Indication that preparticipation screening forms, PAR-Q, and AHA/ACSM Questionnaire were completed
   - Client's current health status and reason for participation
   - Quality and intensity of any pain client is presenting
   - Client's exercise habits
   - Client's medical history including hospitalizations and surgeries
   - Medications or alternative treatments client is taking or receiving, noting frequency and dosage if applicable
   - Client's smoking and alcohol use, if any
   - For women: if client is pregnant and, if so, duration of pregnancy to date

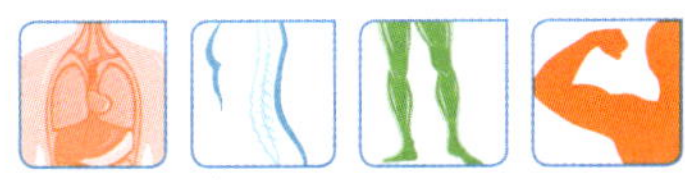

Cardiovascular/Cardiorespiratory Fitness (Part I): *Resting Heart Rate (RHR)*

ITEMS NEEDED: WATCH, STETHOSCOPE (OPTIONAL), HEART RATE MONITOR (OPTIONAL)

1. Client should be seated comfortably for at least 5 minutes.

2. Pulse Palpation: Place first and second fingers over pulse point. For radial pulse, locate near thumbside of wrist. For carotid artery, locate in neck near larynx. Take care to palpate lightly as not to occlude pulse.

3. Auscultation: Place stethoscope left of sternum at level of nipple line.

4. Count pulse rate for 30 seconds and record.

5. Multiply value by 2 to calculate beats per minute. **Refer to Table 1 on page 34 of the workbook and record your calculations using the worksheet on page 34.**

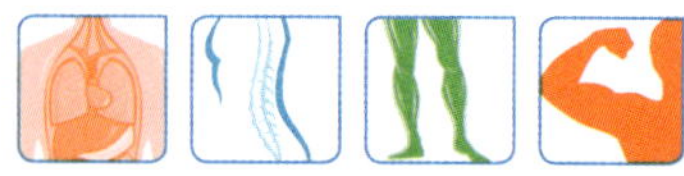

Cardiovascular/Cardiorespiratory Fitness (Part I): *Resting Blood Pressure (RBP)*

ITEMS NEEDED: SPHYGMOMANOMETER, STETHOSCOPE

1. Client should be seated comfortably and allowed to rest for a minimum of 5 minutes. Ingestion of caffeine or nicotine is prohibited 30 minutes prior to test. Client's arms should be bare and supported at level of heart.

2. Wrap cuff firmly around upper arm and align with brachial artery. Appropriate cuff size is required to ensure accurate reading. Bladder within cuff should encircle at least 2/3 of upper arm.

3. Place stethoscope over brachial artery below antecubital space.

4. Inflate cuff to 20 mmHg above estimated systolic blood pressure (SBP).

5. Slowly release cuff pressure at a rate of 2-3 mmHg/s. Note first Korotkoff sound (a).

6. Continue pressure release steadily, note when sound disappears.

7. **Refer to Table 2 on page 34 of the workbook. Using the worksheet on page 34, record first sound (systolic blood pressure, SBP) and pressure at disappearance of sound (diastolic blood pressure, DBP).**

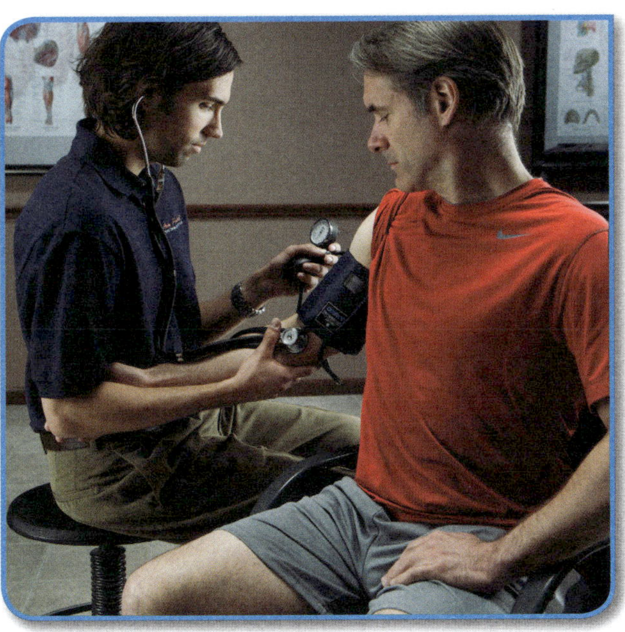

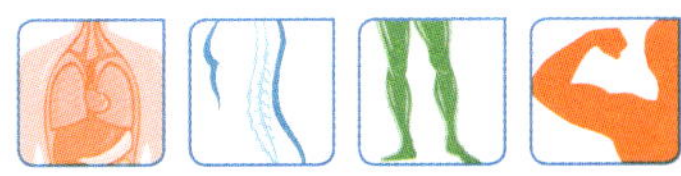

Musculoskeletal Alignment and Development: *Visual Inspection of Posture With Plumb Line*

ITEMS NEEDED: STRING, WEIGHT, TAPE OR EYE HOOK

1. Attach the weight to the string and measure length that spans from ceiling to floor. The weight should just graze the floor and the string should be taut.

2. Hang plumb line from ceiling, preferably 3-4 feet in front of a wall to provide a blank background.

3. Instruct client to disrobe modestly, including shoes and socks.

4. Instruct client to stand between the blank wall and plumb line. Position him or her so line is bisecting most of his or her body. Instruct client to stand comfortably and normally, but be aware that it may take a few minutes for client to exhibit his or her normal habitual posture.

5. Assess posture in anterior (a), lateral (b), and posterior (c) views.

6. **Refer to Figure on page 35 of the workbook.** Note any joint malalignment and significant lack or asymmetry of muscle development, and palpate for bony alignment.

7. **Using the worksheet on page 35, record findings in each view.**

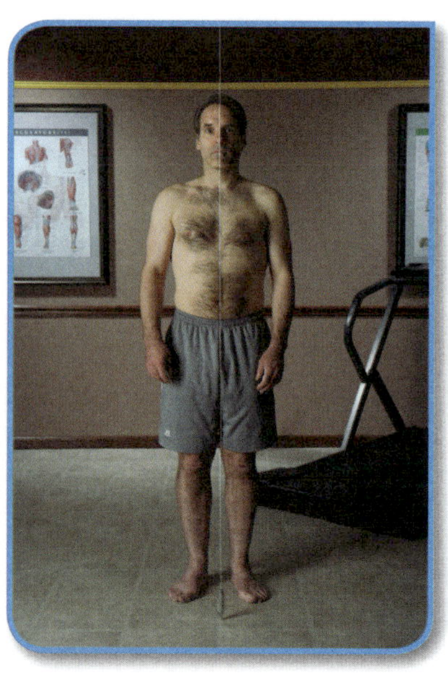

a

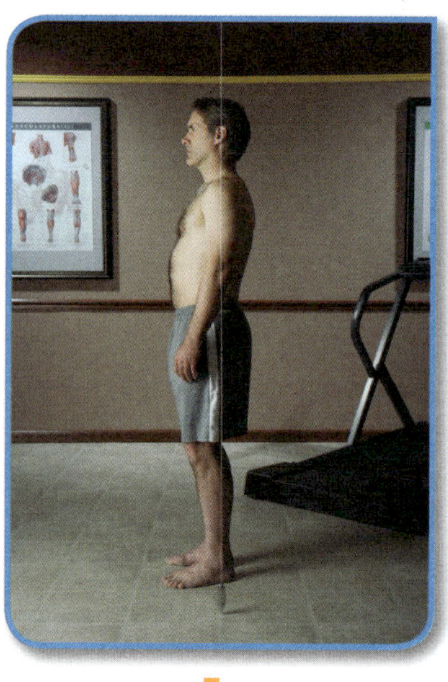

b

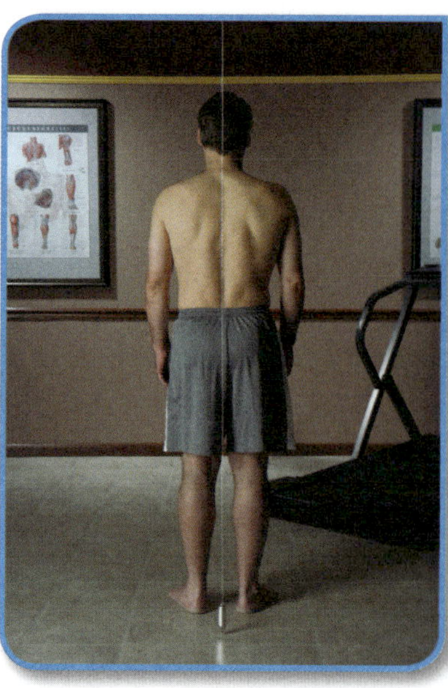

c

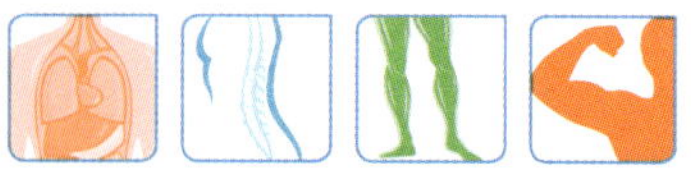

Body Composition: *Body Mass Index and Waist Circumference*

ITEMS NEEDED: SCALE, TAPE MEASURE, MASKING TAPE

1. Instruct client to disrobe modestly, including shoes and socks.

2. Turn scale to "0" and have client step onto scale. Determine his or her weight in pounds (a).

3. Use measuring stick on scale, or fasten tape measure to wall using masking tape. The tape measure should just graze the floor and run perpendicular to it, with the "0" end at the floor. Determine client's height in inches (b).

4. **Using the worksheet on page 36 of the workbook, record values. Refer to Table 4 on page 37 for body mass index (BMI) and record the value.**

5. With client standing in a relaxed position, use the tape measure to measure the portion of the abdomen with the greatest girth (c), which usually is at the level of the umbilicus, in centimeters (cm).

6. **Using the worksheet on page 36, record waist circumference (WC). With BMI value refer to Table 3 on page 36 and record classification of disease risk based on BMI and WC.**

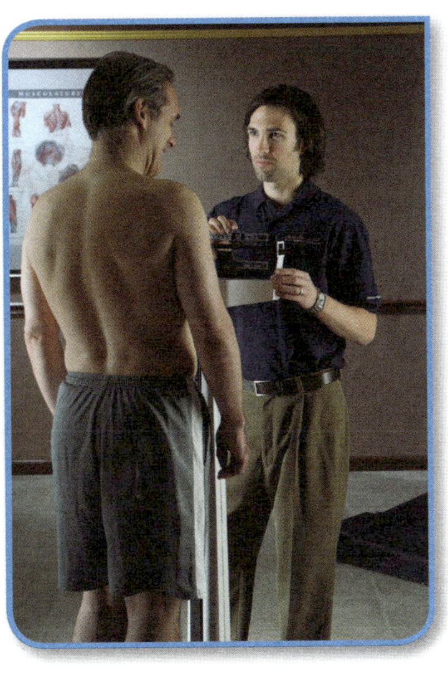

a

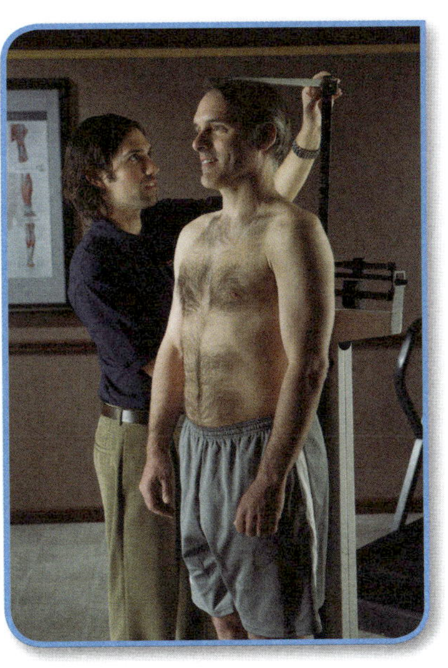

b

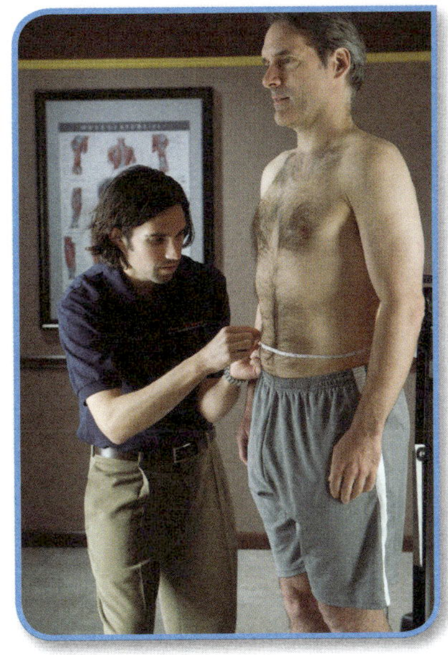

c

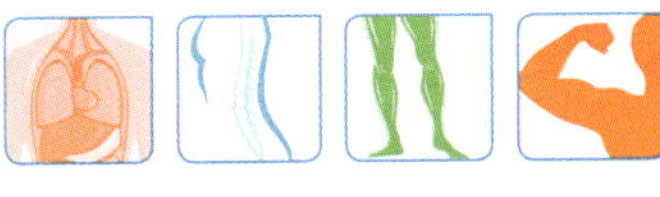

Muscular Flexibility: *Gross Range-of-Motion (ROM) Screen*

ITEMS NEEDED: NONE

1. Use visual inspection to perform a gross body range-of-motion (ROM) screen for upper extremity (neck, shoulder, elbow, wrist, hand); trunk; and lower extremity (hip, knee, ankle, foot).

2. Note and document any ROM deficits. **Refer to Table 5 on page 38 for normative ranges.**

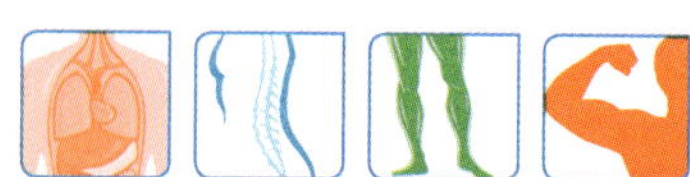

Muscular Flexibility: *Apley's Scratch Test*

ITEMS NEEDED: RULER OR TAPE MEASURE (IF NEEDED)

1. Instruct client to reach over and behind his or her right shoulder with the right upper extremity to touch the left scapula. Say: "Take your right hand and reach for your left shoulder blade as far down your back as possible."

2. Instruct client to then use the left upper extremity to reach behind his or her back from the lower left to touch the fingertips of other hand. Say: "Now with your left hand, reach behind and up your back as far as you can so your fingertips touch" (a).

3. Observe if fingertips touch. **Record Yes or No on page 39 of the workbook. If No, measure distance between fingertips and record to note change over time (b).**

4. Repeat with the opposite upper extremities. Say: "Take your left hand and reach for your right shoulder blade as far down your back as possible. Now with your right hand, reach behind and up your back as far as you can so your fingertips touch" (c).

5. Observe if fingertips touch. **Record Yes or No on page 39 of the workbook. If No, measure distance between fingertips and record to note change over time.**

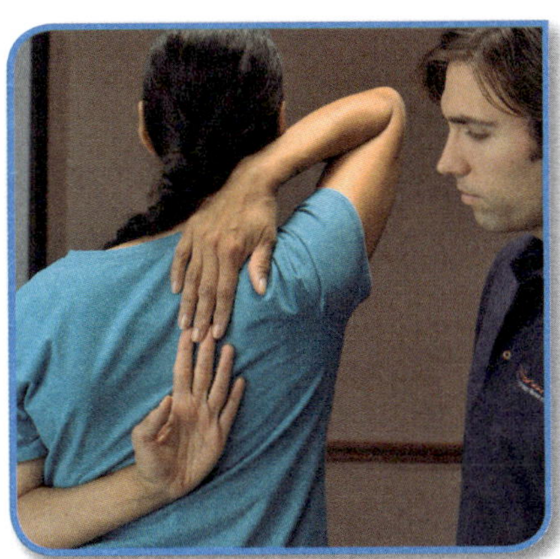

a

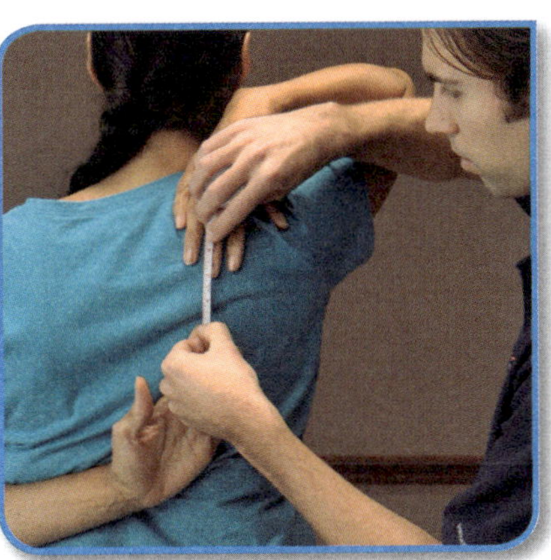

b

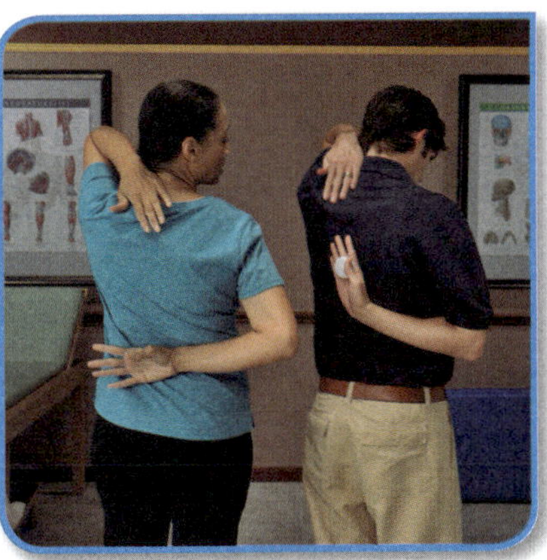

c

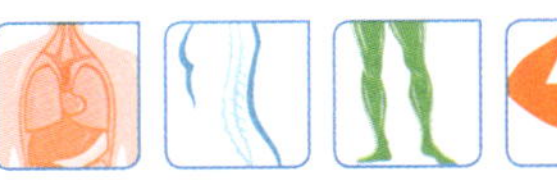

Muscular Flexibility: *YMCA Sit-and-Reach Test*

ITEMS NEEDED: YARDSTICK, MASKING TAPE, MAT (OPTIONAL)

1. Instruct client to warm up with some stretches such as the modified hurdler's stretch. Instruct him or her to refrain from jerky, bouncy movements to avoid injury.

2. Place yardstick on mat or floor, and at the 15-inch mark place approximately 12 inches of masking tape across it, centered at a right angle.

3. Instruct client to sit with yardstick between the legs, legs extended at right angles to the taped line on the floor. Heels of the feet should touch the edge of the taped line and be about 10-12 inches apart (a).

4. Instruct client to slowly reach forward with both hands as far as possible, fingertips extended and in contact with yardstick (b). Client should exhale and drop his or her head between the arms on the way down and hold position momentarily (c).

5. Ensure the knees are in extension and in contact with floor or mat and that client is not performing the Valsalva maneuver.

6. **Using the worksheet on page 39 of the workbook, record the most distant inch-mark on the yardstick reached with the fingertips. Repeat 2 more times.**

7. Use the highest score of the 3 trials, and **refer to Table 6 on page 39 of the workbook to record the appropriate percentile ranking.**

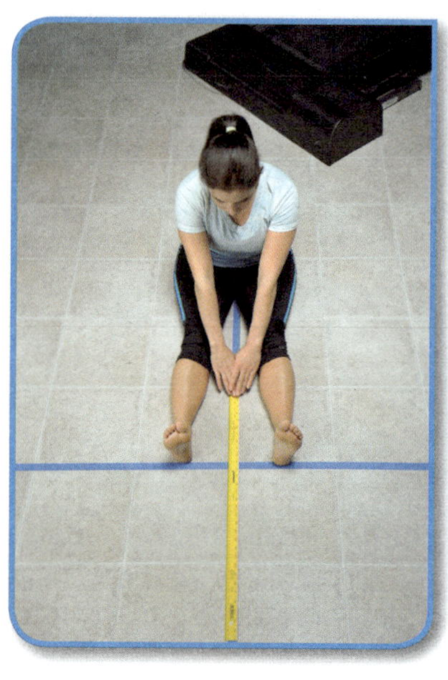
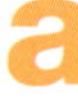

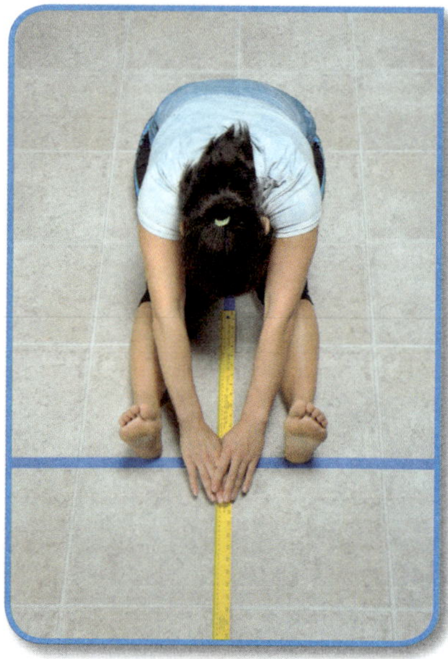

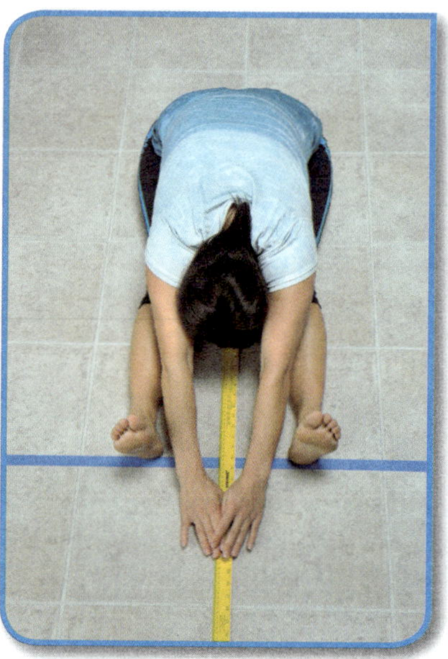
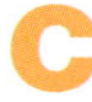

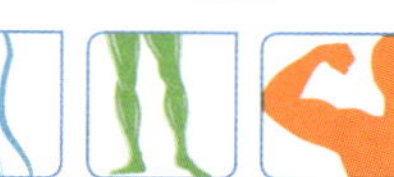

Muscular Strength and Endurance: *Gross Manual Muscle Test (MMT)*

ITEMS NEEDED: NONE

1. Use manually applied break tests to perform a gross manual muscle screen for upper extremity (shoulder, elbow, wrist) and lower extremity (hip, knee, ankle*).
   *Plantarflexion is performed in unilateral stance.

2. **On page 40 of the workbook, note and document any strength deficits.**

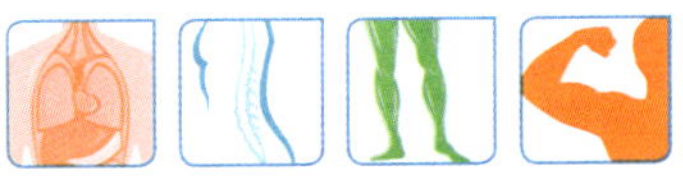

Muscular Strength and Endurance: *Handgrip Strength*

ITEMS NEEDED: HAND DYNAMOMETER

1. Fit dynamometer handgrip comfortably in client's hand with the second joint (PIP) under handle of the dynamometer. **On page 40 of the workbook, note setting (closest, middle, farthest ring).** Reset to zero.

2. Instruct client to hold the dynamometer parallel to the side of his or her body at level of waist. Forearm is to be parallel with the thigh with elbow flexed (a).

3. Instruct client to squeeze handgrip with maximal effort. Take care that he or she does not perform the Valsalva maneuver (b).

4. **Using the worksheet on page 40 of the workbook, record grip strength (kg).** Reset dynamometer to zero.

5. Repeat with opposite hand and **record in the worksheet.** Repeat 2 more times with each hand.

6. **Total the values of the highest recorded strength from each hand (highest left hand value + highest right hand value).** Note a fitness impairment if the combined average is below normal, and/or if there is a difference greater than 10% between the 2 extremities.

7. **Refer to Table 7 on page 40 of the workbook and record the appropriate fitness category.**

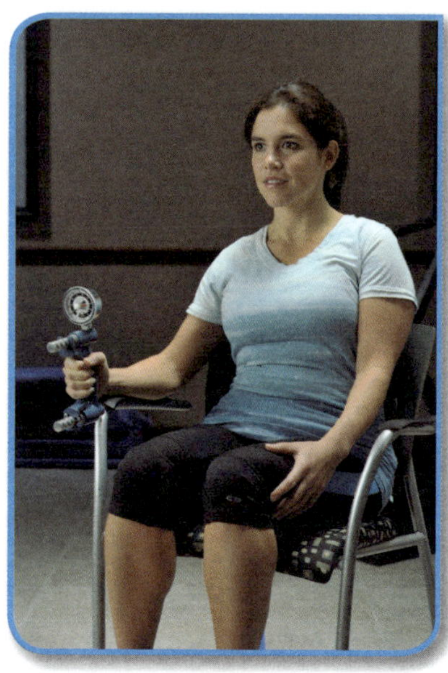

a

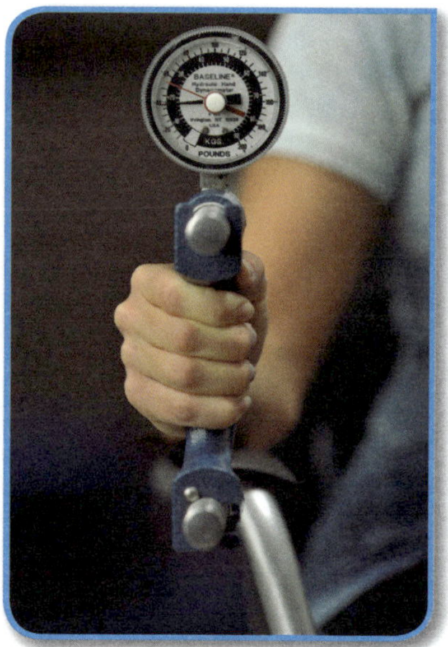

b

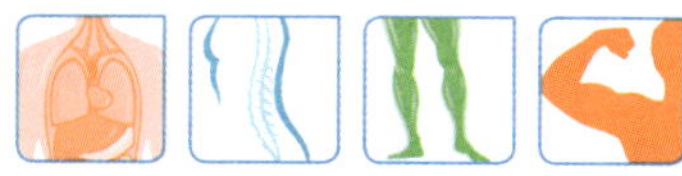

Muscular Strength and Endurance: *Curl-Up (Trunk) Test*

ITEMS NEEDED: METRONOME, MASKING TAPE, RULER OR TAPE MEASURE, MAT (OPTIONAL)

1. Instruct client to lie supine on mat or floor, arms at side with hands flat on the floor, knees at 90°.

2. Place a 6-inch length of masking tape on the floor at the tops of the fingertips of each hand (a).

3. Place a second piece of tape 10 cm beyond the first piece of tape.

4. Set metronome to 50 beats per minute. In time with metronome, have the client perform slow, controlled curl-ups (trunk to about 30° off mat or floor, and fingertips reaching the second piece of tape) with shoulder blades lifted off mat or floor (b) at rate of 25 curl-ups per minute. First beat, curl up; second beat, curl down. Low back should be flattened before next curl-up.

5. Client should perform as many curl-ups as possible up to a maximum of 25.

6. **Using the worksheet on page 41 of the workbook, record number of completed curl-ups. Refer to Table 8 on page 41 and record the appropriate fitness category.**

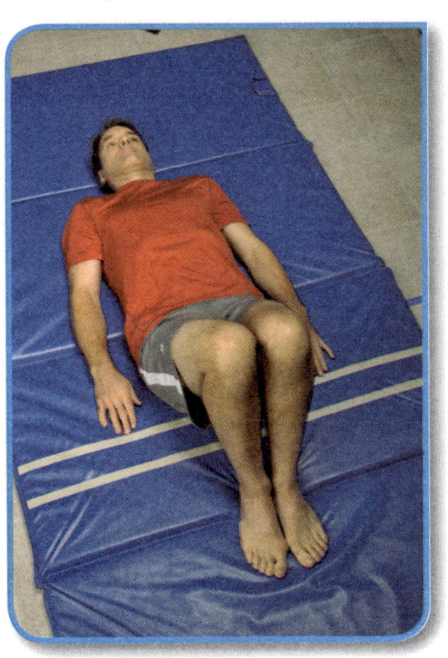

a

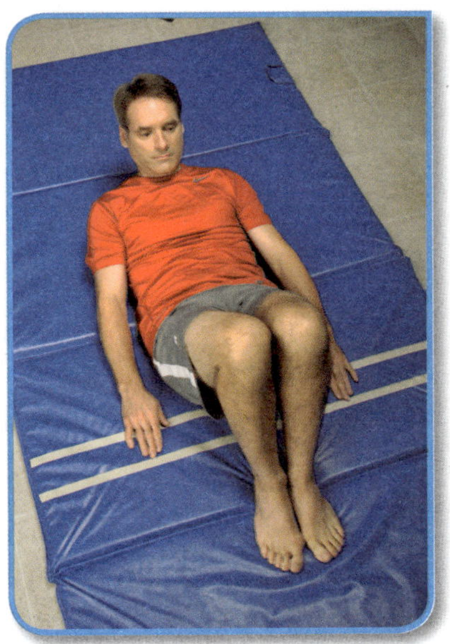

b

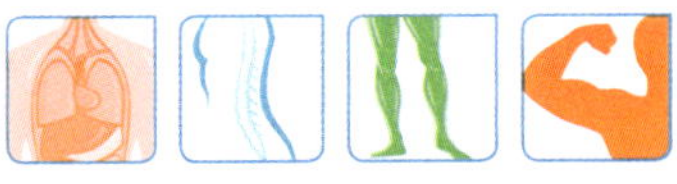

Muscular Strength and Endurance: *Push-Up Test*

ITEMS NEEDED: MAT (OPTIONAL)

1. Position the client for performing push-ups. Men: Standard push-up position—hands shoulder-width apart, back straight, head up, using toes as the pivot point (a). Women: Modified knee push-up—hands shoulder-width apart, back straight, head up, legs together, lower leg lifted from mat or floor, ankles plantarflexed (b).

2. Instruct client to lower his or her body until chin touches mat or floor. Stomach is not to touch mat or floor (c-d, e-f).

3. Client's back and neck must be in straight alignment at all times and push up to a straight arm position.

4. Client should perform as many push-ups as possible without rest, up to 40.

5. **Using the worksheet on page 42 of the workbook, record number of completed push-ups. Refer to Table 9 on page 42 and record the appropriate fitness category.**

a

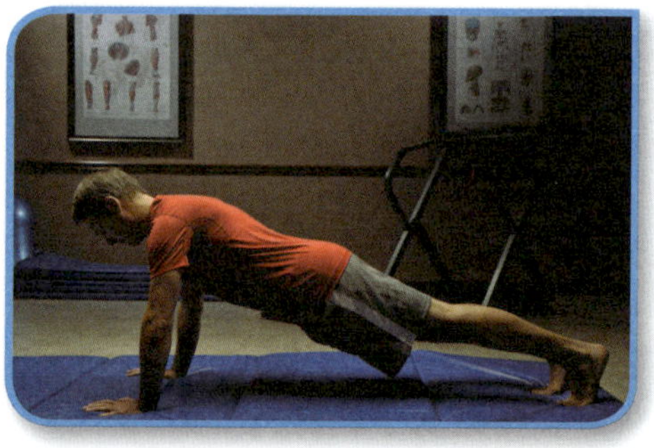

b

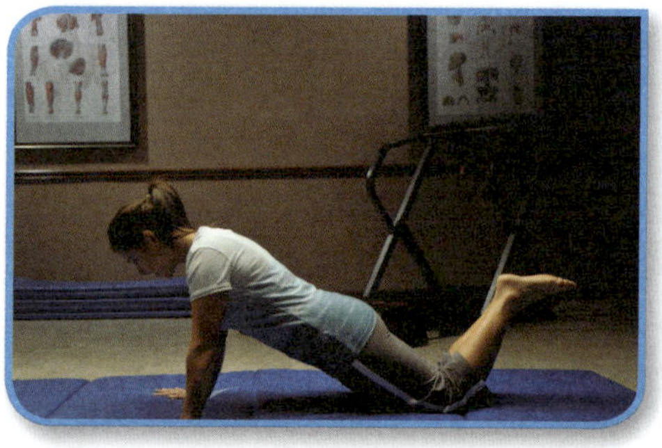

c

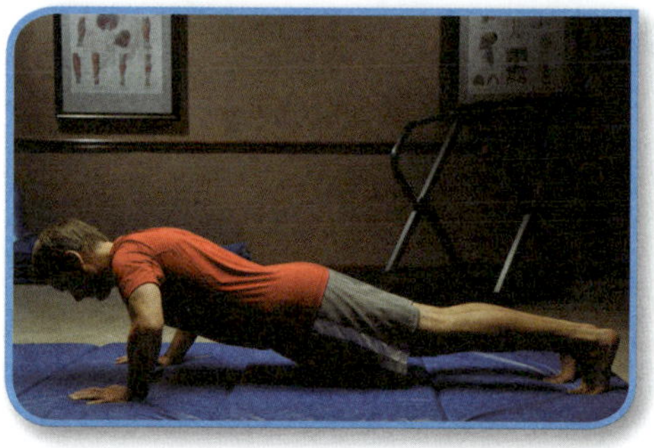

d

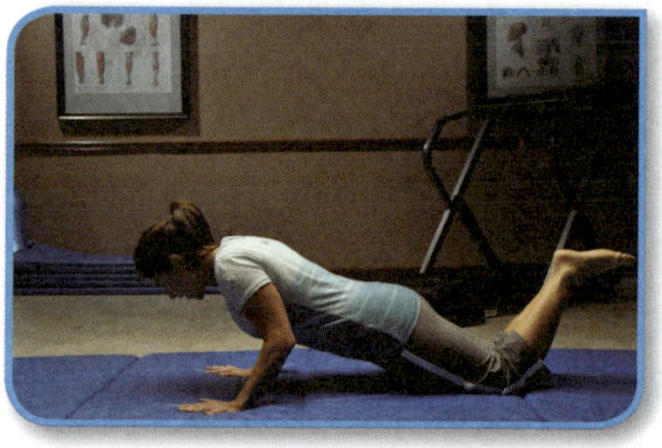

e

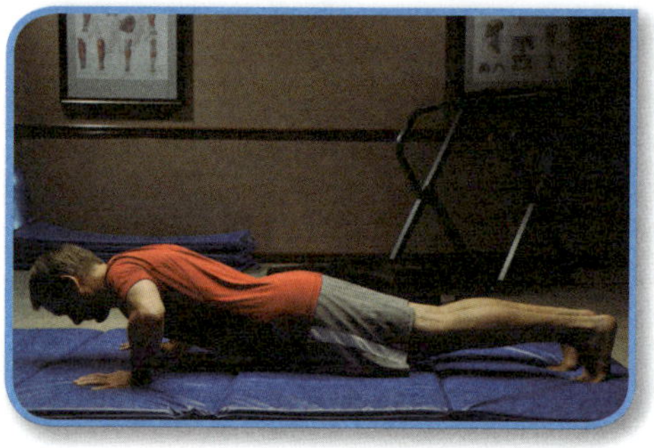

f

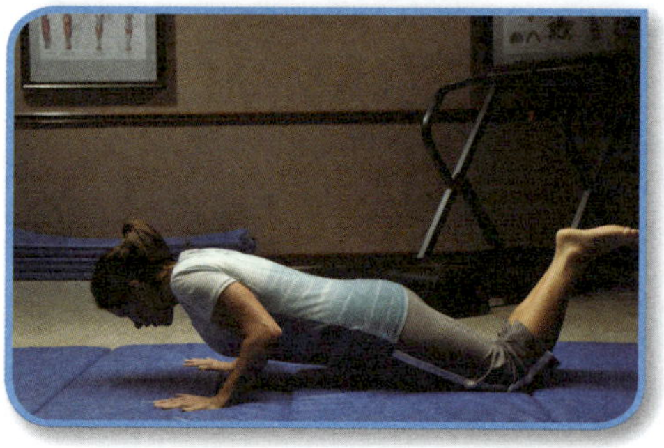

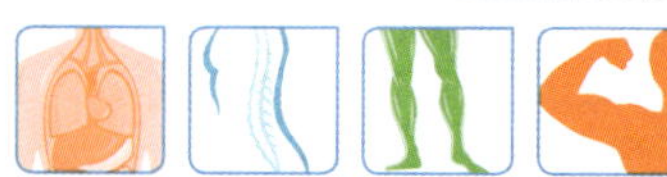

Muscular Strength and Endurance: *Unilateral Step-Down Test*

ITEMS NEEDED: 8-INCH STEP

1. Instruct client to remove shoes and socks and stand with 1 foot on the step and other foot suspended out from the step, unsupported, with bottom of foot level with top of step. Client's arms should be relaxed at the sides but can move during the test to help maintain balance (a).

2. Instruct client to lower the unsupported foot with knee extended, pelvis level to ground, and foot dorsiflexed (b). After touching heel to floor momentarily (c), client should raise his or her foot back up to height of step (a).

3. Client must maintain a straight back and full knee extension of the unsupported leg. Use of hands on thighs is not allowed.

4. Client should complete as many unilateral step-downs as possible, up to 25.

5. Repeat with other leg.

6. **On page 43 of the workbook, record the number of completed repetitions. Refer to Table 10 on page 43 and record the appropriate fitness category.**

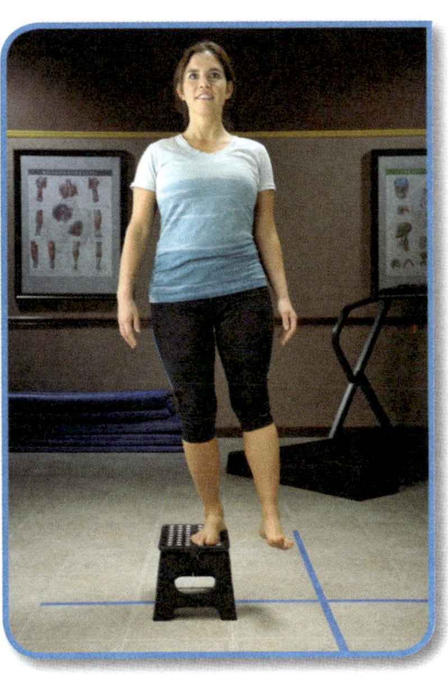
a

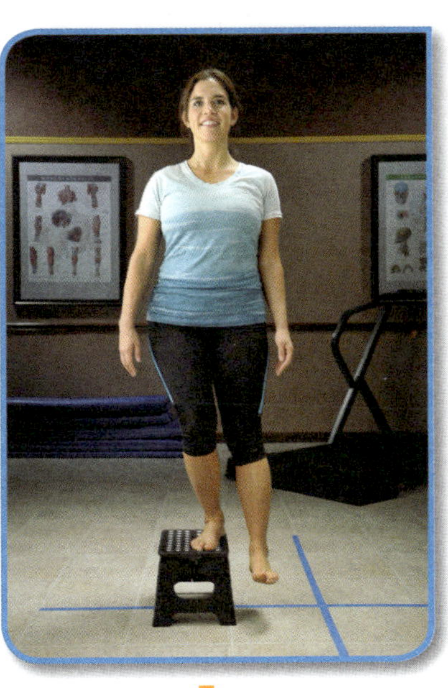
b

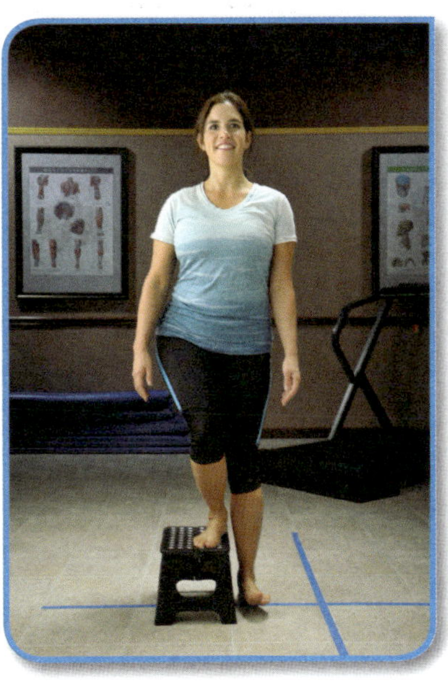
c

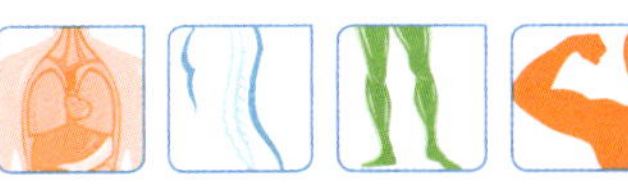

Balance: *Single Limb Stance (SLS) Test*

ITEMS NEEDED: STOPWATCH

1. Instruct client to remove shoes and socks and stand comfortably. Stand nearby in readiness for possible loss of balance.

2. Instruct client to keep eyes open and to stand on 1 leg for as long as possible without losing his or her balance (a). Foot must remain in place. Inform client that testing stops when there is a loss of balance, the other foot touches the floor, or he or she reaches out for support.

3. Say "Start" and start stopwatch. Observe how long client is able to maintain balance. **Using the worksheet on page 44 of the workbook, record up to 90 seconds.**

4. Repeat on other leg. **Record time up to 90 seconds.**

5. Repeat the test on each leg again with client's eyes closed (b), and record times.

6. **Refer to Table 11 on page 44 of the workbook, and record the appropriate fitness category for each leg.** Note that if balance is Above Normative Value with eyes open but Below Normative Value with eyes closed, there may be over-reliance on visual cues, indicating possible limitation in vestibular function.

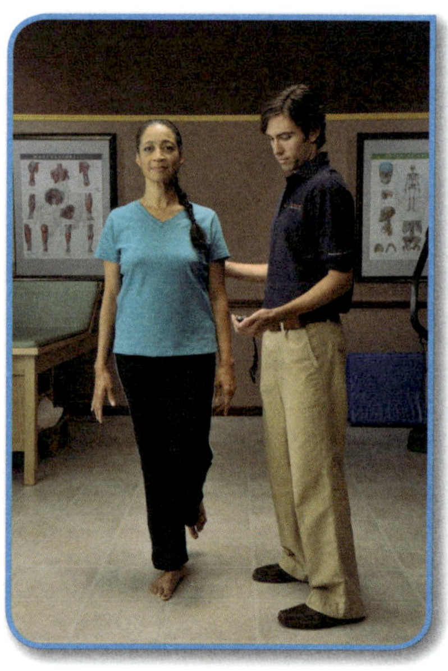

a

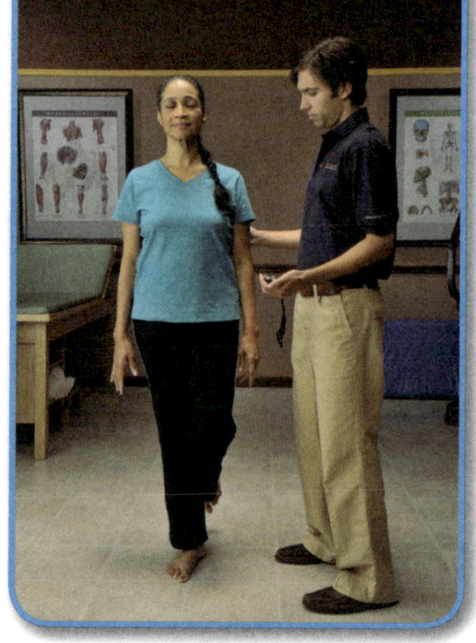

b

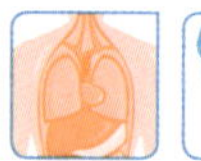
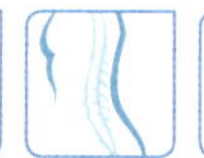
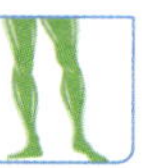

Balance: *Upper Extremity Functional Reach Test*

ITEMS NEEDED: RULER OR TAPE MEASURE, MASKING TAPE

1. Instruct client to remove shoes and socks and stand parallel to wall with dominant upper extremity closest to wall.
2. Affix ruler/tape measure to wall with masking tape at client's shoulder height.
3. Instruct client to make a fist with dominant hand and lift arm parallel to wall (a).
4. **Using the worksheet on page 45, record start position of third metacarpal.**
5. For safety, stand in front and to side of client in case of loss of balance.
6. Instruct client to perform 2 practice forward reaches (b), returning each time to his or her original standing position. Stepping forward or out to the side is not permitted.
7. Instruct client to perform 3 actual trials (c). **Use the worksheet to record ending points for each trial.**
8. Find the difference in distance for each trial and average across three trials.
9. **Refer to Table 12 on page 45 of the workbook, and record the appropriate fitness category.**

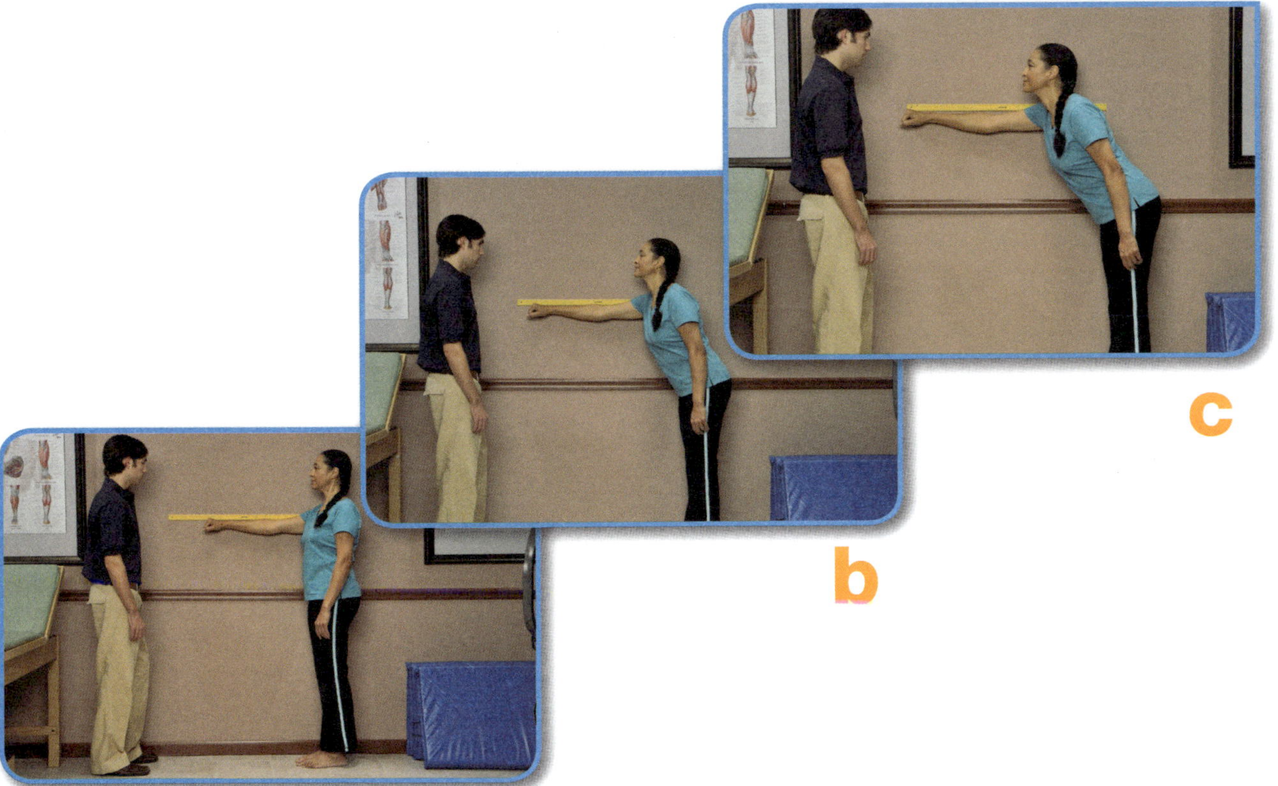

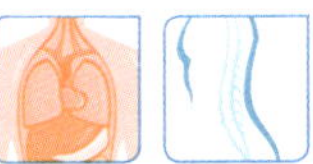
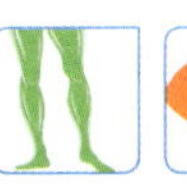

Balance: *Lower Extremity Functional Reach Test*

ITEMS NEEDED: TAPE MEASURE, MASKING TAPE

1. Instruct client to remove shoes and socks and stand. Measure leg length from greater trochanter to lateral malleolus. **Using the worksheet on page 46 of the workbook, record leg lengths for left and right lower extremities.**
2. Mark starting position of big toe of test leg with a piece of masking tape on floor.
3. Instruct client to maintain balance on test leg while reaching as far forward as possible with toe of the other leg, without bearing any weight on toe (a1-2). He or she must be able to return to original standing position without loss of balance. Mark distance with tape. Have client perform 3 trials in forward direction.
4. Repeat in lateral (both left and right, b1-2) and posterior directions (c1-2), 3 trials in each direction.
5. **Using the worksheet on page 46, measure and record farthest distance reached in centimeters (cm) in each direction.**
6. Repeat with opposite leg.
7. Calculate farthest distance reached, divide by length of test leg and multiply by 100 to obtain "percentage of leg length."
8. **Refer to Table 13 on page 46 of the workbook, and record the appropriate fitness category.**

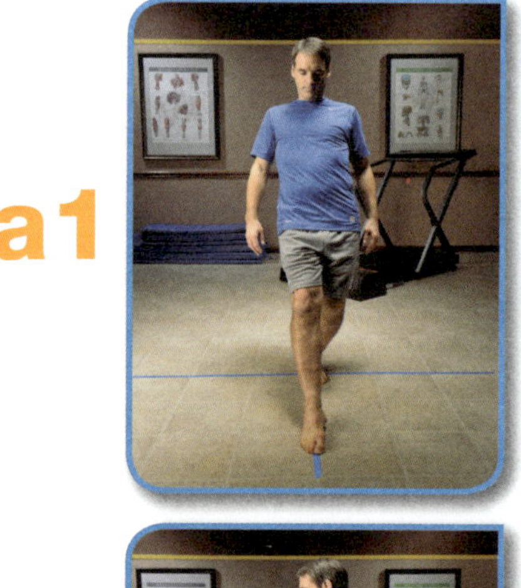
a1

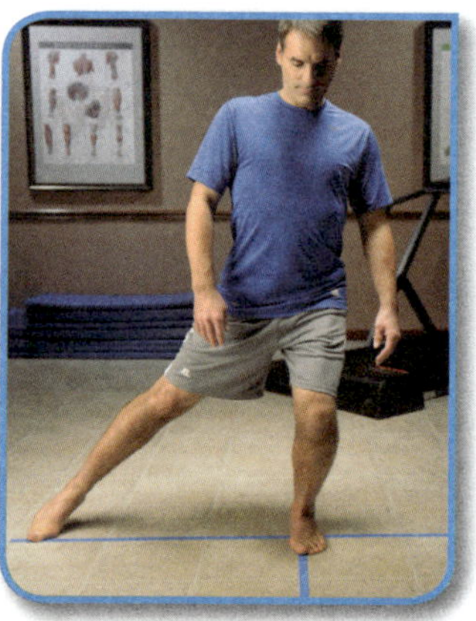
b1

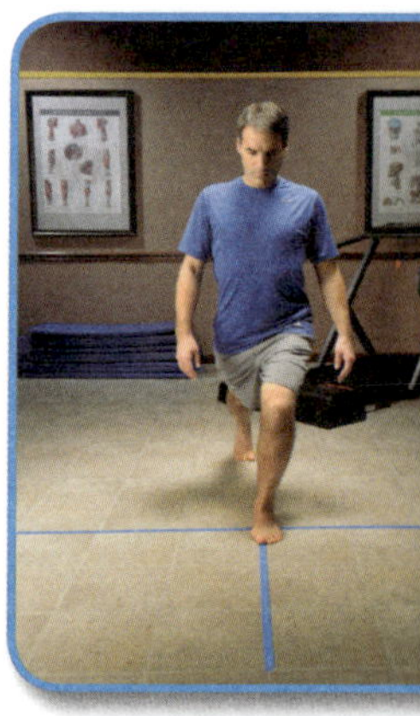
c1

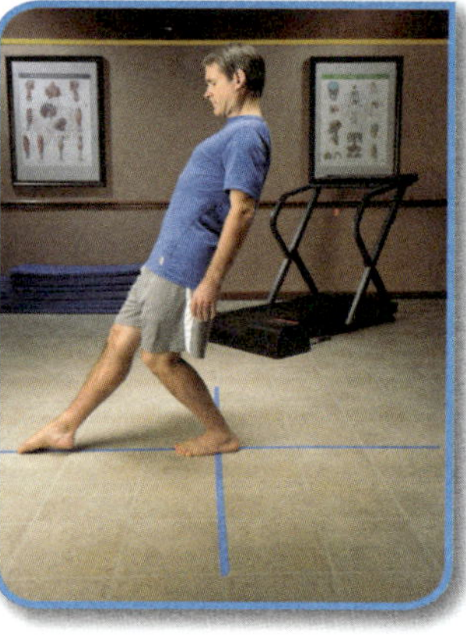
a2

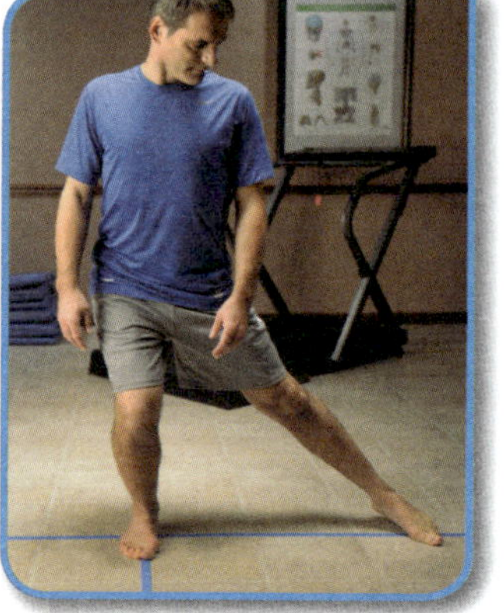
b2

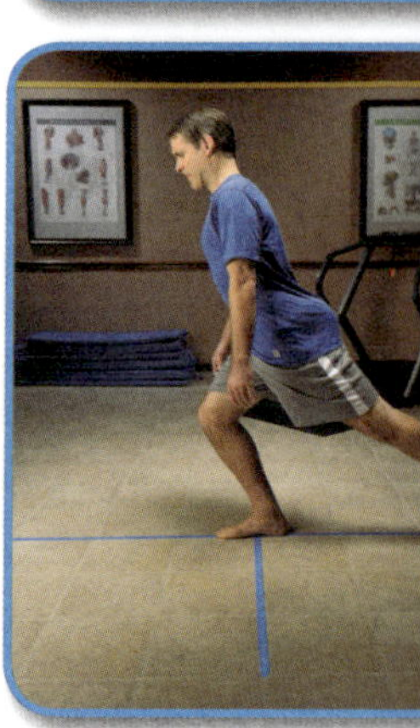
c2

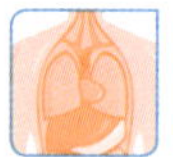 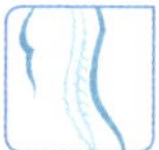 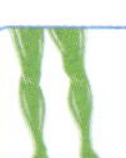 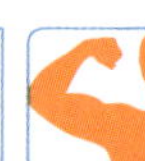

Cardiovascular/Cardiorespiratory Fitness (Part II): *Submaximal Bruce Protocol for Predicted VO2max and Heart Rate Recovery (HRR)*

ITEMS NEEDED: TREADMILL, STOP WATCH, STETHOSCOPE, SPHYGMOMANOMETER, HEART RATE MONITOR (OPTIONAL)

In Preparation: Instruct client on treadmill use and safety. Client should be prepared to walk at least 3 minutes for each stage. Heart rate (HR) will be recorded every minute to determine Heart Rate Steady State (HRss). The previous HR reading must be within 6 bpm to be considered steady state. If client has not reached steady state by the third minute of the stage, he or she is to continue walking at that stage's settings for an additional minute. The HRss should be between 115-155 bpm for the last 2 stages. Blood pressure (BP) should also be recorded during the third minute for each stage.

Important: If patient/client is unable to reach steady-state HR at stage 3, the equation is unable to accurately predict VO2max using SM1 & SM2, as it severely overpredicts, leading to misleading interpretation. VO2max equation should be used only if steady state is reached during stage 3.

Note: Watch for any of these general indications for terminating this test:

- Onset of angina or angina-like symptoms
- Drop of 20 mmHg or greater in SBP or failure of SBP to rise with increase of exercise intensity
- Excessive rise in BP (systolic > 260 or diastolic > 115 mmHg)
- Signs of poor perfusion: lightheadedness, confusion, ataxia, pallor, cyanosis, nausea, or diaphoresis
- Failure of heart rate to increase with increased exercise intensity
- Noticeable change in heart rhythm
- Subject requests to stop
- Physical or verbal manifestations of severe fatigue
- Client reaches 85% of age-predicted maximum heart rate

1. Instruct client to stand facing forward on treadmill. **Determine resting heart rate and blood pressure prior to test and use the Flow Chart for Bruce Protocol on page 48 of the workbook to record.**

2. Say to client: "The test will conclude when you have reached 85% of your maximal heart rate, if you have chest pain, or if you have reached maximum fatigue." Client is not allowed to hold supporting handrails during test.

3. For Stage 1, start treadmill at 1.7 mph and 5% incline for minutes 1 to 3. **Using the Flow Chart for Bruce Protocol, record HR every minute of the stage, and record BP during third minute of the stage (a).**

4. If client is able to continue and HRss is reached, conduct Stage 2 by changing treadmill to 2.5 mph and 12% incline at 4 minutes. **Using the Flow Chart for Bruce Protocol, record HR every minute of the stage, and record BP during third minute of the stage.**

5. If client is unable to reach HRss at the end of Stage 2 within an additional minute, end test. **Make note on the Flow Chart for Bruce Protocol** and inform client that estimate of VO2max cannot be calculated. If client is able to continue and HRss reached, conduct Stage 3 by changing to 3.4 mph and 14% incline at 7 minutes.

6. Conduct Stage 3 until HRss is reached, client complains of chest pain, or client has reached maximum fatigue. If client is unable to reach HRss at the end of Stage 3 within an extra minute, **make note on the Flow Chart for Bruce Protocol** and use Stage 2 findings to calculate predicted VO2max.

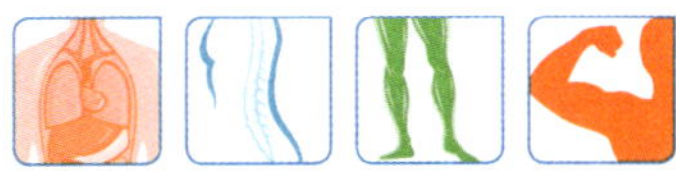

7. As soon as any termination points are encountered, conclude test and have client immediately place feet on sides of treadmill to come to a standing stop. **Using the Flow Chart for Bruce Protocol, take heart rate within 5 seconds and record. Palpate pulse for 15 seconds and record. Also record BP (b).**

8. Multiply heart rate by 4 to calculate peak HR (bpm), and **record on the Flow Chart for Bruce Protocol as "HR end of test."**

9. Two (2) minutes after cessation of the test, reassess HR—take for 15 seconds and **record on the Flow Chart for Bruce Protocol as "HR 2 min after end of test."**

10. To calculate Heart Rate Recovery after 2 minutes (HRR2min): HR end of test - HR 2 min after end of test = HRR2min. **Record HRR2min in the worksheet on page 48.**

11. **Refer to Table 14 on page 49 to record the appropriate fitness category.**

12. **Refer to *Predicting VO2max From Submaximal Bruce Protocol Results* on page 48, and input data into the appropriate formula on page 47.**

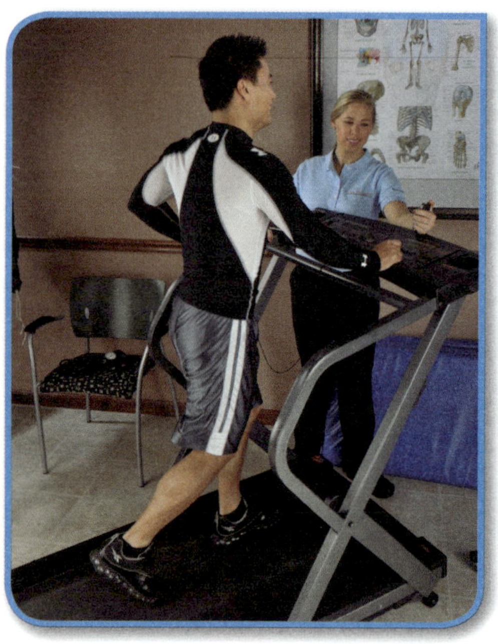

a

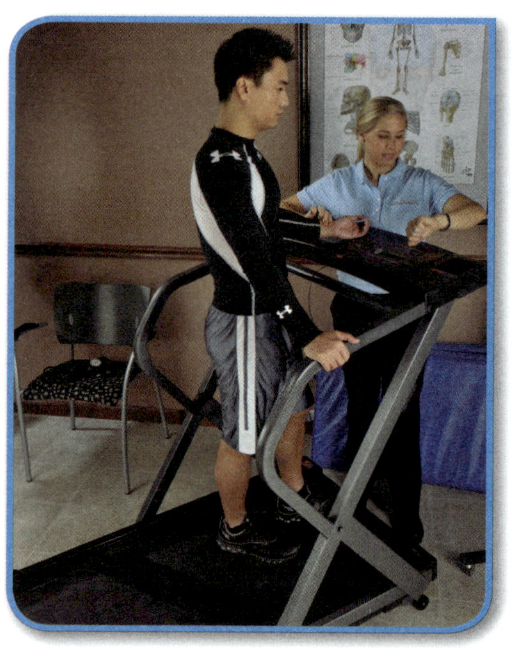

b

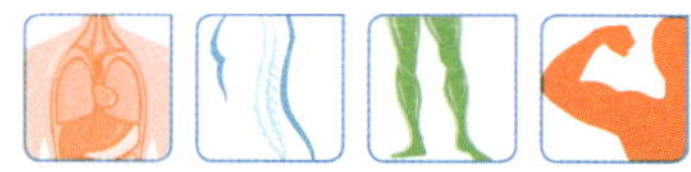

Adult Fitness Examination: Workbook

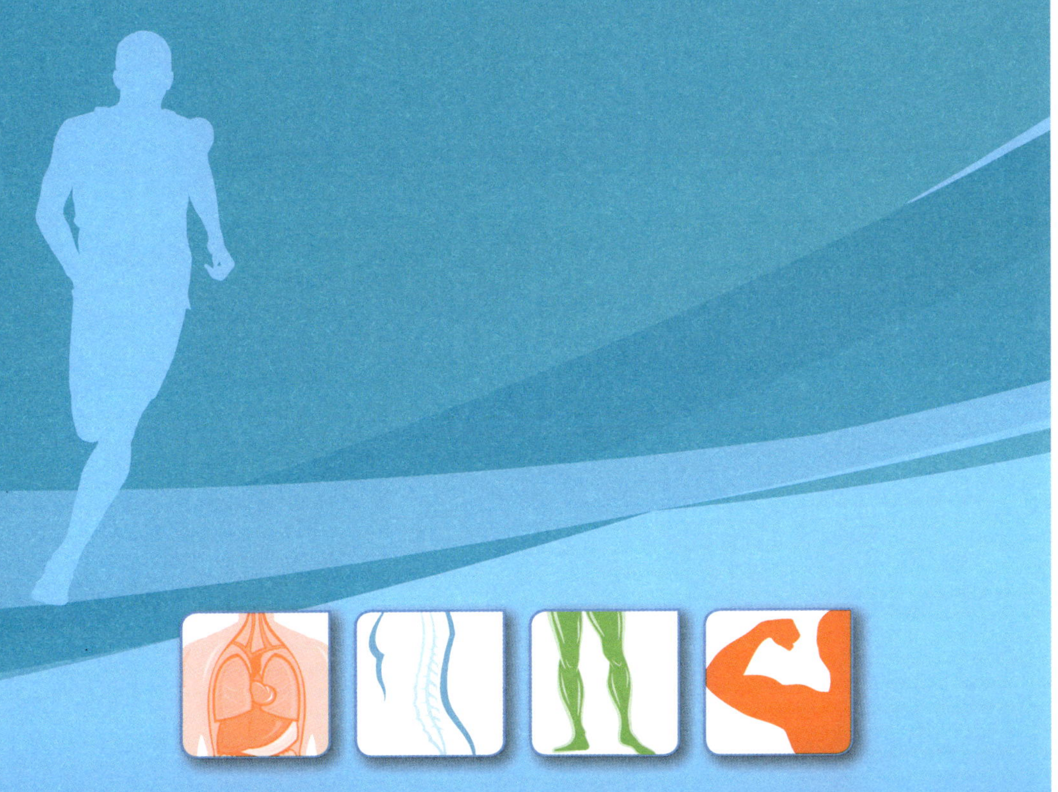

Preparticipation Health Screening: *Physical Activity Readiness Questionnaire (PAR-Q)*

Physical Activity Readiness Questionnaire - PAR-Q (revised 2002)

PAR-Q & YOU

(A Questionnaire for People Aged 15 to 69)

Regular physical activity is fun and healthy, and increasingly more people are starting to become more active every day. Being more active is very safe for most people. However, some people should check with their doctor before they start becoming much more physically active.

If you are planning to become much more physically active than you are now, start by answering the seven questions in the box below. If you are between the ages of 15 and 69, the PAR-Q will tell you if you should check with your doctor before you start. If you are over 69 years of age, and you are not used to being very active, check with your doctor.

Common sense is your best guide when you answer these questions. Please read the questions carefully and answer each one honestly: check YES or NO.

YES	NO	
☐	☐	**1. Has your doctor ever said that you have a heart condition and that you should only do physical activity recommended by a doctor?**
☐	☐	**2. Do you feel pain in your chest when you do physical activity?**
☐	☐	**3. In the past month, have you had chest pain when you were not doing physical activity?**
☐	☐	**4. Do you lose your balance because of dizziness or do you ever lose consciousness?**
☐	☐	**5. Do you have a bone or joint problem (for example, back, knee or hip) that could be made worse by a change in your physical activity?**
☐	☐	**6. Is your doctor currently prescribing drugs (for example, water pills) for your blood pressure or heart condition?**
☐	☐	**7. Do you know of any other reason why you should not do physical activity?**

If you answered

YES to one or more questions

Talk with your doctor by phone or in person BEFORE you start becoming much more physically active or BEFORE you have a fitness appraisal. Tell your doctor about the PAR-Q and which questions you answered YES.

- You may be able to do any activity you want — as long as you start slowly and build up gradually. Or, you may need to restrict your activities to those which are safe for you. Talk with your doctor about the kinds of activities you wish to participate in and follow his/her advice.
- Find out which community programs are safe and helpful for you.

NO to all questions

If you answered NO honestly to all PAR-Q questions, you can be reasonably sure that you can:

- start becoming much more physically active – begin slowly and build up gradually. This is the safest and easiest way to go.
- take part in a fitness appraisal – this is an excellent way to determine your basic fitness so that you can plan the best way for you to live actively. It is also highly recommended that you have your blood pressure evaluated. If your reading is over 144/94, talk with your doctor before you start becoming much more physically active.

DELAY BECOMING MUCH MORE ACTIVE:

- if you are not feeling well because of a temporary illness such as a cold or a fever – wait until you feel better; or
- if you are or may be pregnant – talk to your doctor before you start becoming more active.

PLEASE NOTE: If your health changes so that you then answer YES to any of the above questions, tell your fitness or health professional. Ask whether you should change your physical activity plan.

Informed Use of the PAR-Q: The Canadian Society for Exercise Physiology, Health Canada, and their agents assume no liability for persons who undertake physical activity, and if in doubt after completing this questionnaire, consult your doctor prior to physical activity.

No changes permitted. You are encouraged to photocopy the PAR-Q but only if you use the entire form.

NOTE: If the PAR-Q is being given to a person before he or she participates in a physical activity program or a fitness appraisal, this section may be used for legal or administrative purposes.

"I have read, understood and completed this questionnaire. Any questions I had were answered to my full satisfaction."

NAME ______________________

SIGNATURE ______________________ DATE ______________________

SIGNATURE OF PARENT ______________________ WITNESS ______________________
or GUARDIAN (for participants under the age of majority)

Note: This physical activity clearance is valid for a maximum of 12 months from the date it is completed and becomes invalid if your condition changes so that you would answer YES to any of the seven questions.

continued on other side...

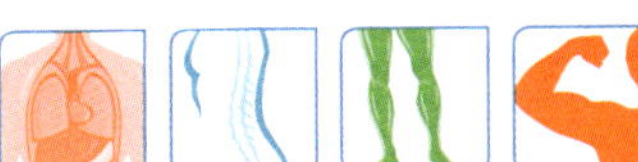

Preparticipation Health Screening: *AHA/ACSM Health/ Fitness Facility Preparticipation Screening Questionnaire*

ASSESS YOUR HEALTH NEEDS BY MARKING ALL TRUE STATEMENTS.

History

You have had:

- ○ A heart attack
- ○ Heart surgery
- ○ Cardiac catheterization
- ○ Coronary angioplasty (PTCA)
- ○ Pacemaker/implantable cardiac defibrillator/rhythm disturbance
- ○ Heart valve disease
- ○ Heart failure
- ○ Heart transplant
- ○ Congenital heart disease

Symptoms

- ○ You experience chest discomfort with exertion.
- ○ You experience unreasonable breathlessness.
- ○ You experience dizziness, fainting, blackouts.
- ○ You take heart medication(s).

Other health issues

- ○ You have diabetes.
- ○ You have asthma or other lung disease.
- ○ You have burning or cramping in your lower legs when walking short distances.
- ○ You have musculoskeletal problems that limit your physical ability.
- ○ You have concerns about the safety of exercise.
- ○ You take prescription medication(s).
- ○ You are pregnant.

If you marked any of the statements in these sections, consult your physician or other appropriate health care provider before participation.

Cardiovascular risk factors

- ○ You are a man older than 45 years.
- ○ You are a woman older than 55 years, have had a hysterectomy, or are postmenopausal.
- ○ You smoke, or you quit within the previous 6 months.
- ○ Your blood pressure is greater than 140/90 mmHg.
- ○ You don't know your blood pressure.
- ○ You take blood pressure medication.
- ○ Your blood cholesterol level is >200 mg/dL.
- ○ You don't know your blood cholesterol level.
- ○ You have a close blood relative who had a heart attack before age 55 (father or brother) or age 65 (mother or sister).
- ○ You are physically inactive (ie, you get <30 minutes of physical activity at least 3 days per week).
- ○ You are more than 20 pounds overweight.

If you marked two or more of the statements in this section, you should consult your physician or other appropriate health care provider before participation.

- ○ None of the above is true.

You should be able to participate safely without consulting your physician.

Adapted with permission from: American College of Sports Medicine Position Stand and American Heart Association. Recommendations for cardiovascular screening, staffing, and emergency policies at health/fitness facilities. *Med Sci Sport Exerc*. 1998;30(6):1009-1018.

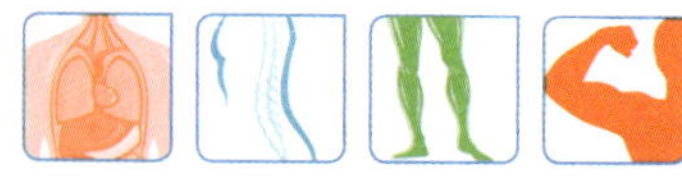

Preparticipation Health Screening: *Client Information*

Client Name: ______________________________ Date of AFE: ______________

Age: __________ Sex: ○ Male ○ Female Hand Dominance: ○ Right ○ Left

PAR-Q and AHA/ACSM Preparticipation Screening Questionnaire Completed: ○ Yes ○ No

Current Overall Health Status: ______________________________

____

____

____

____

Pain? Location: ______________ Type: ______________ Intensity: ______/10

Physically Active: ○ Yes ○ No If Yes, Frequency/Duration/Intensity: ______________

Type(s) of Activity(ies): ______________________________

Past Medical History/Hospitalizations/Surgeries: ______________________________

____

____

____

____

Medications/Vitamins/Supplements: ______________________________

____

____

____

____

HEALTH ISSUES

Smoking: Currently: ○ No ○ Yes If Yes, Frequency __________

History: ○ No ○ Yes If Yes, Frequency __________ # of Years __________

Alcohol: Currently: ○ No ○ Yes If Yes, Frequency __________

History: ○ No ○ Yes If Yes, Frequency __________ # of Years __________

Pregnancy: Currently: ○ No ○ Yes If Yes, Weeks along __________

History: Number of pregnancies __________

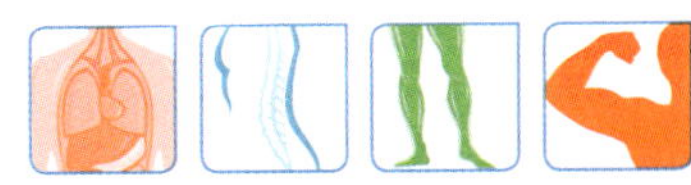

Cardiovascular/Cardiorespiratory Fitness (Part I): *Resting Heart Rate (RHR)*

________ (pulse rate for 30 seconds) × 2 = ________ bpm = RHR

Fitness Category (refer to Table 1): ○ Bradycardia ○ Normal ○ Tachycardia

Table 1. Ranges for Resting Heart Rate (RHR)

CATEGORY	RESTING HEART RATE (BPM)
Bradycardia	< 60*
Normal	60–100
Tachycardia	> 100

*Well-trained healthy individuals can exhibit normal RHR of 30–50 bpm.

Adapted from: Rothstein JM, Roy SH, Wolf SL. *The Rehabilitation Specialist's Handbook*. 3rd ed. Philadelphia, PA: F. A. Davis Company; 2005. McArdle W, Katch F, Katch V. *Exercise Physiology: Energy, Nutrition, and Human Performance*. 5th ed. Philadelphia, PA: Lippincott Williams & Wilkins; 2001.

Resting Blood Pressure (RBP)

________ SBP (mmHg) / ________ DBP (mmHg)

Fitness Category (refer to Table 2): ○ Normal ○ Prehypertension ○ Stage 1 ○ Stage 2

Table 2. Classification of Blood Pressure for Adults Aged 18 and Older

CATEGORY	SYSTOLIC BP, mmHg (SBP)		DIASTOLIC BP, mmHg (DBP)
Normal	< 120	AND	< 80
Prehypertension	120–139	OR	80–89
HYPERTENSION			
Stage 1	140–159	OR	90–99
Stage 2	> 160	OR	> 100

From: NBHLI. *JNC VIII Express: The Seventh Report of the Joint National Committee on Prevention, Detection, Evaluation, and Treatment of High Blood Pressure*. Washington, DC: National Blood, Heart and Lung Institute, National Institutes of Health; 2003:19.

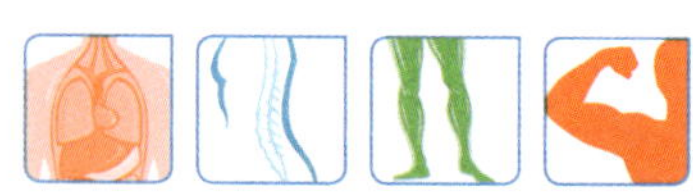

Musculoskeletal Alignment and Development: *Visual Inspection of Posture With Plumb Line*

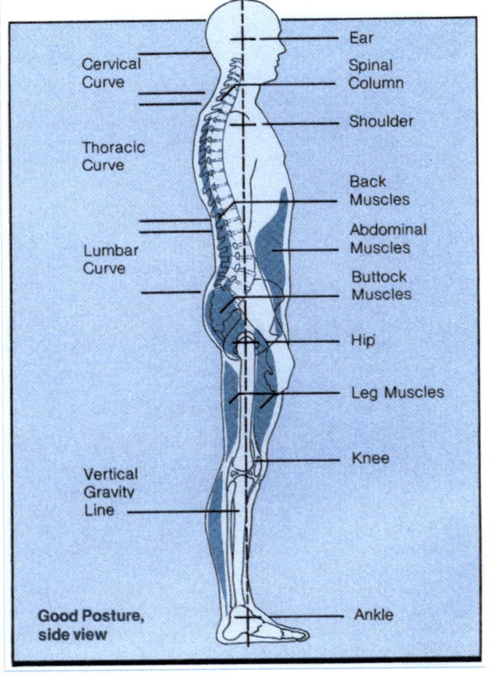

Good Posture, side view

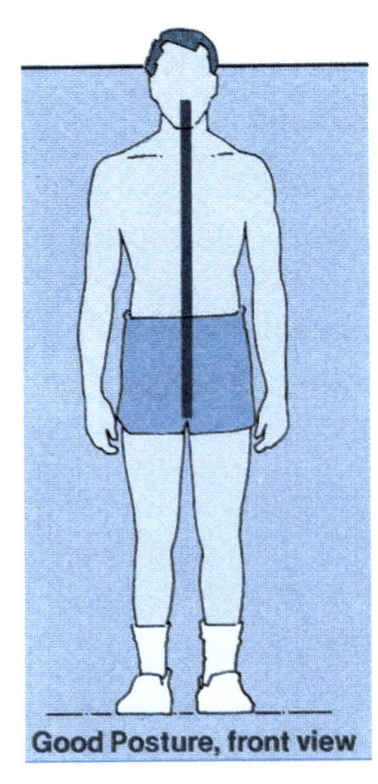

Good Posture, front view

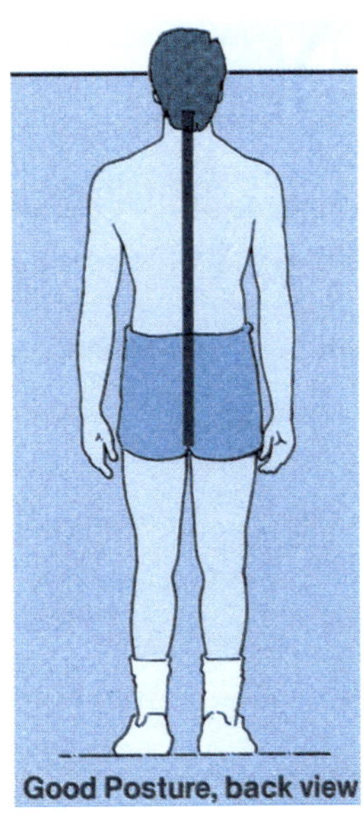

Good Posture, back view

Notes:

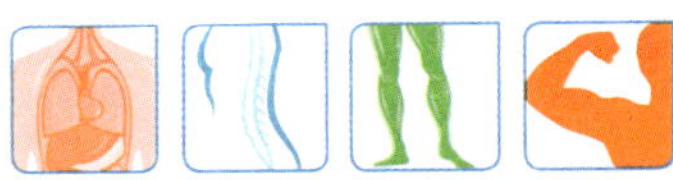

Body Composition: *Body Mass Index (BMI) and Waist Circumference (WC)*

Height = ________ inches Weight = ________ pounds Waist Circumference (WC) = ________ inches

BMI (refer to Table 4, page 37) = ________ (________ cm)

Classification based on BMI and WC (refer to Table 3): ○ Underweight ○ Normal ○ Overweight ○ Obesity, Class I ○ Obesity, Class II ○ Obesity, Class III

Table 3. Classification of Disease Risk Based on Body Mass Index (BMI) and Waist Circumference (WC)

Disease Risk Relative to Normal Weight and WC

	BMI (per Table 4)	WC: MEN, ≤102 CM (40 IN) WC: WOMEN, ≤88 CM (35 IN)	WC: MEN, >102 CM (40 IN) WC: WOMEN, >88 CM (35 IN)
Underweight	<18.5	...	...
Normal	18.5–24.9	...	...
Overweight	25.0–29.9	Increased	High
Obesity, Class I	30.00–34.9	High	Very high
Obesity, Class II	35.0–39.9	Very high	Very high
Obesity, Class III	≥40.0	Extremely high	Extremely high

Adapted from: National Heart, Lung and Blood Institute. Executive Summary of the clinical guidelines on the Identification, Evaluation, and Treatment of Overweight and Obesity in Adults. Washington, DC: National Heart, Lung and Blood Institute of the National Institutes of Health. http://www.nhlbi.nih.gov/guidelines/obesity/ob_gdlns.htm. Accessed September 21, 2009.

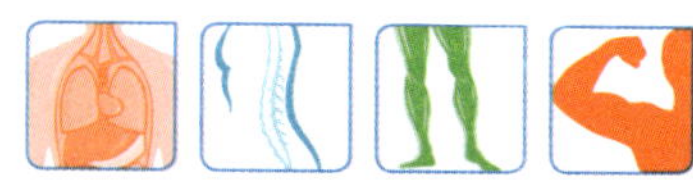

Table 4. Body Mass Index

Body Mass Index Table

	Normal						Overweight					Obese										Extreme Obesity														
BMI	**19**	**20**	**21**	**22**	**23**	**24**	**25**	**26**	**27**	**28**	**29**	**30**	**31**	**32**	**33**	**34**	**35**	**36**	**37**	**38**	**39**	**40**	**41**	**42**	**43**	**44**	**45**	**46**	**47**	**48**	**49**	**50**	**51**	**52**	**53**	**54**
Height (inches)																Body Weight (pounds)																				
58	91	96	100	105	110	115	119	124	129	134	138	143	148	153	158	162	167	172	177	181	186	191	196	201	205	210	215	220	224	229	234	239	244	248	253	258
59	94	99	104	109	114	119	124	128	133	138	143	148	153	158	163	168	173	178	183	188	193	198	203	208	212	217	222	227	232	237	242	247	252	257	262	267
60	97	102	107	112	118	123	128	133	138	143	148	153	158	163	168	174	179	184	189	194	199	204	209	215	220	225	230	235	240	245	250	255	261	266	271	276
61	100	106	111	116	122	127	132	137	143	148	153	158	164	169	174	180	185	190	195	201	206	211	217	222	227	232	238	243	248	254	259	264	269	275	280	285
62	104	109	115	120	126	131	136	142	147	153	158	164	169	175	180	186	191	196	202	207	213	218	224	229	235	240	246	251	256	262	267	273	278	284	289	295
63	107	113	118	124	130	135	141	146	152	158	163	169	175	180	186	191	197	203	208	214	220	225	231	237	242	248	254	259	265	270	278	282	287	293	299	304
64	110	116	122	128	134	140	145	151	157	163	169	174	180	186	192	197	204	209	215	221	227	232	238	244	250	256	262	267	273	279	285	291	296	302	308	314
65	114	120	126	132	138	144	150	156	162	168	174	180	186	192	198	204	210	216	222	228	234	240	246	252	258	264	270	276	282	288	294	300	306	312	318	324
66	118	124	130	136	142	148	155	161	167	173	179	186	192	198	204	210	216	223	229	235	241	247	253	260	266	272	278	284	291	297	303	309	315	322	328	334
67	121	127	134	140	146	153	159	166	172	178	185	191	198	204	211	217	223	230	236	242	249	255	261	268	274	280	287	293	299	306	312	319	325	331	338	344
68	125	131	138	144	151	158	164	171	177	184	190	197	203	210	216	223	230	236	243	249	256	262	269	276	282	289	295	302	308	315	322	328	335	341	348	354
69	128	135	142	149	155	162	169	176	182	189	196	203	209	216	223	230	236	243	250	257	263	270	277	284	291	297	304	311	318	324	331	338	345	351	358	365
70	132	139	146	153	160	167	174	181	188	195	202	209	216	222	229	236	243	250	257	264	271	278	285	292	299	306	313	320	327	334	341	348	355	362	369	376
71	136	143	150	157	165	172	179	186	193	200	208	215	222	229	236	243	250	257	265	272	279	286	293	301	308	315	322	329	338	343	351	358	365	372	379	386
72	140	147	154	162	169	177	184	191	199	206	213	221	228	235	242	250	258	265	272	279	287	294	302	309	316	324	331	338	346	353	361	368	375	383	390	397
73	144	151	159	166	174	182	189	197	204	212	219	227	235	242	250	257	265	272	280	288	295	302	310	318	325	333	340	348	355	363	371	378	386	393	401	408
74	148	155	163	171	179	186	194	202	210	218	225	233	241	249	256	264	272	280	287	295	303	311	319	326	334	342	350	358	365	373	381	389	396	404	412	420
75	152	160	168	176	184	192	200	208	216	224	232	240	248	256	264	272	279	287	295	303	311	319	327	335	343	351	359	367	375	383	391	399	407	415	423	431
76	156	164	172	180	189	197	205	213	221	230	238	246	254	263	271	279	287	295	304	312	320	328	336	344	353	361	369	377	385	394	402	410	418	426	435	443

From: National Heart, Lung and Blood Institute. Body Mass Index Table. Washington, DC: National Heart, Lung and Blood Institute of the National Institutes of Health. http://www.nhlbi.nih.gov/guidelines/obesity/bmi_tbl.htm. Accessed September 18, 2009.

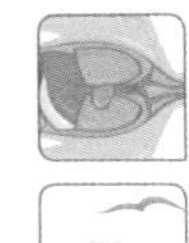
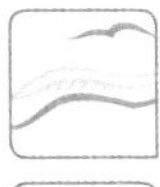
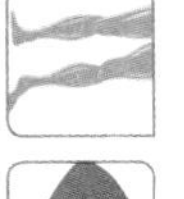

Muscular Flexibility: *Gross Range-of-Motion (ROM) Screen*

List Findings:

Cervical ROM:

Upper Extremities:

Lower Extremities:

Table 5. Normative Values[a] for Range of Motion for Adults Per Various Authors (in degrees, except for TMJ)

AREA	AAOS	KENDALL ET AL	HIRSCH ET AL
NECK (CERVICAL MOVEMENT)			
Flexion	0-45	45-50*	
Extension	0-45	45-75*	
Lateral flexion	0-45	45-60*	
Rotation	0-60	60-80*	
MOUTH (TMJ)			
Opening			51 mm
Left lateral excursion			10-11 mm
Right lateral excursion			10 mm
Protrusion			8 mm
SHOULDER			
Flexion	0-180	180	
Extension	0-60	45	
Abduction	0-180	180	
Horizontal abduction		90	
Horizontal adduction	0-135	40	
Internal (medial) rotation	0-70	70	
External (lateral) rotation	0-90	90	
LUMBAR SPINE	80	80	
ELBOW/FOREARM			
Flexion/extension	0-150	145	
Supination	0-80	90	
Pronation	0-80	90	
WRIST/HAND			
Flexion	0-80	80	
Extension	0-70	70	
Ulnar deviation	0-30	35	
Radial deviation	0-20	20	
THUMB			
CMC flexion	0-15	15	
CMC extension	0-20	20	
CMC abduction	0-70	60	
CMC opposition		Pad of thumb to pad of 5th digit	
MCP flexion	0-50	50	
MCP extension	0	0	
IP flexion	0-80	80	
IP extension	0-20	0	

AREA	AAOS	KENDALL ET AL	HIRSCH ET AL
Digits 2-5			
MCP flexion	0-90	90	
MCP extension	0-45	0	
MCP abduction		20	
PIP flexion	0-100	100	
PIP extension	0	0	
DIP flexion	0-90	70	
DIP extension		0	
HIP			
Flexion	0-120	125	
Extension	0-30	10	
Abduction	0-45	45	
Adduction	0-30	10	
Internal rotation	0-45	45	
External rotation	0-45	45	
KNEE			
Flexion/extension	0-135	140	
ANKLE/FOOT			
Dorsiflexion	0-20	20	
Plantar flexion	0-50	45	
Inversion	0-35	40	
Eversion	0-15	20	
TOE			
Flexion	30		
Extension	40		

[a]Published "norms" for range of motion vary widely; the AFE has compiled ranges from 3 sources for reference.

Adapted with permission from: *Joint Motion: Method of Measuring and Recording.* Chicago: American Academy of Orthopedic Surgeons; 1965. Kendall FP, McCreary EK, Provance PG, Rodgers MM, Romani WA. *Muscles: Testing and Function.* 5th ed. Baltimore, MD: Lippincott, Williams & Wilkins; 2005. Hirsch C, John MT, Lautenschlager C, List T. Mandibular jaw movement capacity in 10-17-yr-old children and adolescents: normative values and the influence of gender, age, and tempromandibular disorders. *Eur J Oral Sci.* 2006;114:465-470.

*Kendall figures are compiled from these sources: Palmer ML, Epler ME. *Fundamentals of Musculoskeletal Assessment Techniques.* 2nd ed. Philadelphia: Lippincott; 1998:221-224. Clarkson HM. *Musculoskeletal Assessment.* 2nd ed. Baltimore: Lippincott Williams & Wilkins; 2000:402. Reese NB, Bandy WD. *Joint Range of Motion and Muscle Length Testing.* Philadelphia: WB Saunders; 2002:408.

Muscular Flexibility: *Apley's Scratch Test*

Do client's fingers touch in mid back? :

Right arm overhead, left arm behind back: ○ Yes ○ No If No, distance between fingertips ________ cm

Left arm overhead, right arm behind back: ○ Yes ○ No If No, distance between fingertips ________ cm

Muscular Flexibility: *YMCA Sit-and-Reach Test*

	FARTHEST DISTANCE REACHED (IN)
Trial 1	
Trial 2	
Trial 3	
Best of 3 trials	

Percentile Ranking for YMCA Sit-and-Reach (refer to Table 6): ○ 10 ○ 20 ○ 30 ○ 40 ○ 50 ○ 60 ○ 70 ○ 80 ○ 90

Table 6. Percentiles by Age Groups and Sex for YMCA Sit-and-Reach Test (inches)

PERCENTILE	AGE AND SEX									
	18–25		26–35		36–45		46–55		56–65	
	M	F	M	F	M	F	M	F	M	F
90	22	24	21	23	21	22	19	21	17	20
80	20	22	19	21	19	21	17	20	15	19
70	19	21	17	20	17	19	15	18	13	17
60	18	20	17	20	16	18	14	17	13	16
50	17	19	15	19	15	17	13	16	11	15
40	15	18	14	17	13	16	11	14	9	14
30	14	17	13	16	13	15	10	14	9	13
20	13	16	11	15	11	14	9	12	7	11
10	11	14	9	13	7	12	6	10	5	9

Reprinted with permission from: *Physical Fitness Assessments and Norms for Adults and Law Enforcement.* Dallas, TX: The Cooper Institute; 2009. http://www.cooperinstitute.org.

Muscular Strength and Endurance: *Gross Manual Muscle Test (MMT)*

Upper Extremities:

Lower Extremities:

Muscular Strength and Endurance: *Handgrip Strength*

Handgrip Ring Setting: ○ Closest ○ Middle ○ Farthest

	LEFT ○ (check if dominant)	RIGHT ○ (check if dominant)	% difference between hands*
Trial 1			
Trial 2			
Trial 3			
Highest value			
Sum of both hands (kg)			

* Difference of more than 10% indicates fitness impariment

Combined Grip Strength Rating (refer to Table 7): ○ Above Average ○ Average ○ Below Average ○ Poor

Table 7. Normative Ranges for Handgrip Strength by Age Groups and Sex for Combined Right and Left Hand

GRIP STRENGTH (kg)	AGE AND SEX					
	15–19		20–29		30–39	
	M	F	M	F	M	F
Above average	103–112	64–70	113–123	65–70	113–122	66–72
Average	95–102	59–63	106–112	61–64	105–112	61–65
Below average	84–94	54–58	97—105	55–60	97–104	56–60
Poor	≤ 83	≤ 53	≤ 96	≤ 54	≤ 96	≤ 55

GRIP STRENGTH (kg)	AGE AND SEX					
	45–49		50–59		60–69	
	M	F	M	F	M	F
Above average	110–118	62–72	102–109	59–64	98–101	54–69
Average	102–109	59–64	96–101	55–58	86–97	51–53
Below average	94–101	55–58	87—95	51–54	79–85	48–50
Poor	≤ 93	≤ 54	≤ 86	≤ 54	≤ 78	≤ 47

Reprinted with permission from: American College of Sports Medicine. *Health-Related Physical Fitness Assessment Manual.* 2005:75.

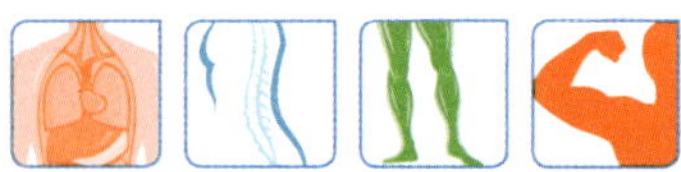

Muscular Strength and Endurance: *Curl-Up (Trunk) Test*

Number of curl-ups completed: __________ reps

Fitness Category (refer to Table 8): ○ Excellent ○ Very Good ○ Good ○ Fair ○ Needs Improvement

Table 8. Fitness Categories by Age Groups and Sex for Partial Curl-Ups

CATEGORY	AGE AND SEX									
	20–29		30–39		40–49		50–59		60–69	
	M	F	M	F	M	F	M	F	M	F
Excellent	25	25	25	25	25	25	25	25	25	25
Very Good	24	24	24	24	24	24	24	24	24	24
	21	18	18	19	18	19	17	19	16	17
Good	20	17	17	18	17	18	16	18	15	16
	16	14	15	10	13	11	11	10	11	8
Fair	15	13	14	9	6	4	4	6	6	3
	11	5	11	6	6	4	4	6	6	3
Needs Improvement	10	4	10	5	5	3	3	5	5	2

From: Canadian Physical Activity, Fitness & Lifestyle Approach: CSEP-Health & Fitness Program's Health-related Appraisal & Counseling Strategy. 3rd ed. 2003. Adapted with permission from the Canadian Society for Exercise Physiology.

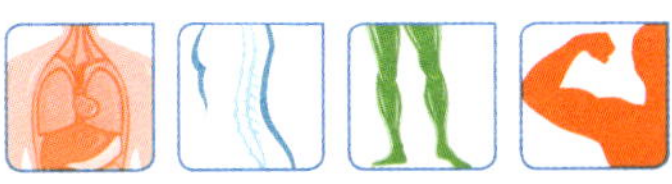

Muscular Strength and Endurance: *Push-Up Test*

Number of push-ups completed: __________ reps

Fitness Category (refer to Table 9): ○ Excellent ○ Very Good ○ Good ○ Fair ○ Needs Improvement

Table 9. Fitness Categories by Age Groups and Sex for Push-Ups

CATEGORY	AGE AND SEX									
	20–29		30–39		40–49		50–59		60–69	
	M	F	M	F	M	F	M	F	M	F
Excellent	36	30	30	27	25	24	21	21	18	17
Very Good	35	29	29	26	24	23	20	20	17	16
	29	21	22	20	17	15	13	11	11	12
Good	28	20	21	19	16	14	12	10	10	11
	22	15	17	13	13	11	10	7	8	5
Fair	21	14	16	12	12	10	9	6	7	4
	17	10	12	8	10	5	7	2	5	2
Needs Improvement	16	9	11	7	9	4	6	1	4	1

From: Canadian Physical Activity, Fitness & Lifestyle Approach: CSEP-Health & Fitness Program's Health-related Appraisal & Counseling Strategy. 3rd Ed. 2003. Adapted with permission from the Canadian Society for Exercise Physiology.

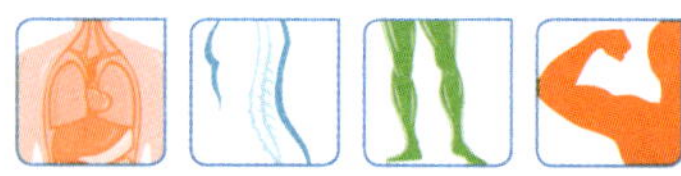

ʌluscular Strength and Endurance: Jnilateral Step-Down Test

ɪumber of step-downs completed:

eft: ______ reps Fitness Category (refer to Table 10): ○ Normal ○ Good ○ Fair ○ Poor ○ Unable

ight: _____ reps Fitness Category (refer to Table 10): ○ Normal ○ Good ○ Fair ○ Poor ○ Unable

able 10. Fitness Categories for the Unilateral Step-Down Test

Normal	20 or more reps
Good	15–19 reps
Fair	10–14 reps
Poor	1–9 reps
Unable	0 reps

rom: Chua A. Physical therapy assessment of adult fitness: a prospective protocol. [unpublished manuscript] Valhalla, NY: New York Medical College;)05. Slovin S, Millrood D. Criterion-referenced data for functional lower extremity strength testing. [unpublished manuscript] Valhalla, NY: New York ɪedical College; 2006. McGann T, Millrood D. Criterion-referenced data for functional lower extremity strength testing. [unpublished manuscript] alhalla, NY: New York Medical College; 2007.

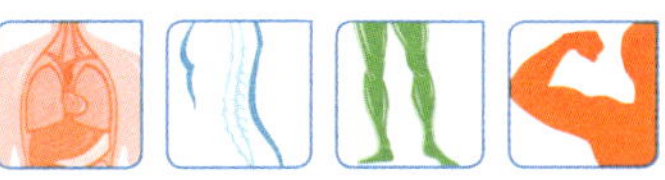

Balance: *Single Limb Stance (SLS) Test*

	STANCE TIME ON LEFT LEG (sec)	STANCE TIME ON RIGHT LEG (sec)
Eyes open		
Eyes closed		

SLS balance on LEFT leg, eyes open (refer to Table 11): O Below Normative Value O Above Normative Value

SLS balance on LEFT leg, eyes closed (refer to Table 11): O Below Normative Value O Above Normative Value

SLS balance on RIGHT leg, eyes open (refer to Table 11): O Below Normative Value O Above Normative Value

SLS balance on RIGHT leg, eyes closed (refer to Table 11): O Below Normative Value O Above Normative Value

Note: If balance is Above Normative Value with eyes open but Below Normative Value with eyes closed, there may be over-reliance on visual cues, indicating possible limitation in vestibular function.

Table 11. Normative Values for Single Limb (Unipedal) Stance by Age Groups and Sex for Eyes Open and Closed

CATEGORY	EYES OPEN, AGE AND SEX (sec) MEAN (SE)							
	18–39		40–49		50–59		60–69	
	M	F	M	F	M	F	M	F
Best of 3 Trials	44.4 (4.1)	45.1 (0.1)	41.6 (10.2)	42.1 (9.5)	41.5 (10.5)	40.9 (10.0)	33.8 (16.0)	30.4 (16.4)

CATEGORY	EYES CLOSED, AGE AND SEX (sec) MEAN (SE)							
	18–39		40–49		50–59		60–69	
	M	F	M	F	M	F	M	F
Best of 3 Trials	16.9 (13.9)	13.1 (12.3)	12.0 (13.5)	13.5 (12.4)	8.6 (8.8)	7.9 (8.0)	5.1 (6.8)	3.6 (2.3)

From: Springer B, Marin R, Cyhan T, et al. Normative values for the Unipedal Stance Test with eyes open and closed. *J Geria Phys Ther.* 2007;30(1):11.

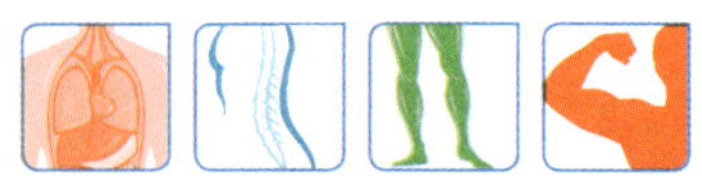

alance: *Upper Extremity Functional Reach Test*

	TRIAL 1 (INCHES)	TRIAL 2 (INCHES)	TRIAL 3 (INCHES)
tarting point (3rd metacarpal)			
nding point (3rd metacarpal)			
istance reached (start – end)			

ial 1 ________ + Trial 2 ________ + Trial 3 = ________ /3 = ________ **Average reaching distance**

per Extremity Functional Reach (refer to Table 12):

Below Normative Range ○ Within Normative Range ○ Above Normative Range

ble 12. Normative Ranges for Upper Extremity Functional Reach Test

AGE AND SEX			
20–40		41–69	
M	F	M	F
16.2 ± 1.9 in.	14.6 ± 2.2 in.	14.9 ± 2.2 in.	13.8 ± 2.2 in.

m: Duncan PW, Weiner DK, Chadler J, Studenske S. Functional reach: a new clinical measure of balance. *J Gerontol.* 1990;45:M192. Used with nission from the Gerontological Society of America and Oxford University Press.

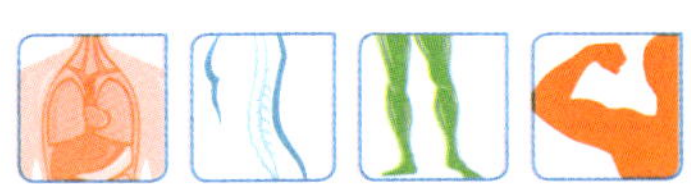

Balance: *Lower Extremity Functional Reach Test*

Length of leg (greater trochanter to lateral malleolus):

Left lower extremity = ________ cm   Right lower extremity = ________ cm

Left Lower Extremity

	DISTANCE REACHED (CM)	DIVIDE	LEG LENGTH (CM)	× 100	% OF LEG LENGTH	FITNESS CATEGORY (REFER TO TABLE 13)
Anterior		/		=		
Lateral		/		=		
Posterior		/		=		

Right Lower Extremity

	DISTANCE REACHED (CM)	DIVIDE	LEG LENGTH (CM)	× 100	% OF LEG LENGTH	FITNESS CATEGORY (REFER TO TABLE 13)
Anterior		/		=		
Lateral		/		=		
Posterior		/		=		

Lower Extremity Functional Reach (refer to Table 13): ○ Normal ○ Good ○ Fair ○ Poor

Table 13. Fitness Categories for Lower Extremity Functional Reach Test

	ANTERIOR REACH	LATERAL REACH	POSTERIOR REACH
Normal	>/=80% leg length	>/=100% leg length	>/=110% leg length
Good	70-79% leg length	90-99% leg length	95-109% leg length
Fair	65-69% leg length	80-89% leg length	85-94% leg length
Poor	<65% leg length	<80% leg length	<85% leg length

From: Slovin S, Millrood D. Criterion-referenced data for functional lower extremity strength testing. [unpublished manuscript] Valhalla, NY: New York Medical College; 2006. McGann T, Millrood D. Criterion-referenced data for functional lower extremity strength testing. [unpublished manuscript] Valhalla, NY: New York Medical College; 2007.

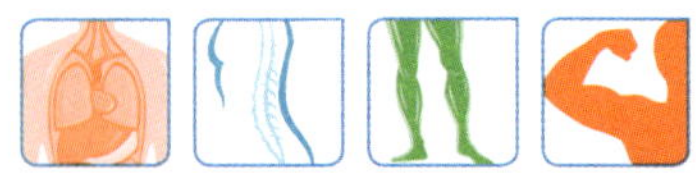

Cardiovascular/Cardiorespiratory Fitness (Part II): *Submaximal Bruce Protocol for Predicted VO2max and Heart Rate Recovery (HRR)*

PREDICTING VO2MAX FROM SUBMAXIMAL BRUCE PROTOCOL RESULTS

Calculate the slope of the HR and V02 relationship and then calculate the V02max using the slope.

Important: *If patient/client is unable to reach steady-state HR at stage 3, the equation is unable to accurately predict VO2max using SM1 & SM2; it severly overpredicts leading to misleading interpretation. VO2max equation should be used only if steady state is reached during stage 3.*

1. For treadmill walking (1.9-3.7 mph):

Submaximal predicted VO2 (SM) = $[(m^*min^{-1}) \times 0.1] + [(m^*min^{-1}) \times 1.8 \times \text{grade (decimal)}] + 3.5\ mL^*\ kg^{-1}{}^*min^{-1}$

Speed conversion: 1 mph = $26.8\ m^*min^{-1}$

2. If client reached HRss in Stage 3:

SM2 = $24.6\ mL^*kg^{-1}{}^*min^{-1}$

SM3 = $35.5\ mL^*kg^{-1}{}^*min^{-1}$

Determine the slope (b) of the HR and VO2:

$$b = \frac{(SM3-SM2)}{(HR3-HR2)} = \frac{(35.5 - 24.6)}{(HR3-HR2)} = \frac{(10.9)}{(HR3-HR2)}$$

Where:

SM2 = Submaximal predicted VO2 from stage 2

SM3 = Submaximal predicted VO2 from stage 3

HR2 = Steady state HR in bpm, from stage 2

HR3 = Steady state HR in bpm, from stage 3

3. Predicted VO2max = SM3 + b (HRmax – HR3)

Where: HRmax = 220 - age

4. Refer to Table 15 on page 49 for the appropriate sex.

5. HRR2min from flow chart (refer to Table 14 on page 49):

- O Excellent
- O Good
- O Average
- O Fair
- O Poor

Adapted with permission from: Vehrs PR, George JD, Fellingham GW, Plowman SA, Dustman-Allen K. Submaximal treadmill exercise test to predict VO2max in fit adults. *Meas Phys Ed Exerc Sci.* 2007;11:2,61-72. Bruce RA, Kusumi F, Hosmer D. Maximal oxygen intake and nomographic assessment of functional aerobic impairment in cardiovascular disease. *Am Heart J.* 1973;85:546–562.

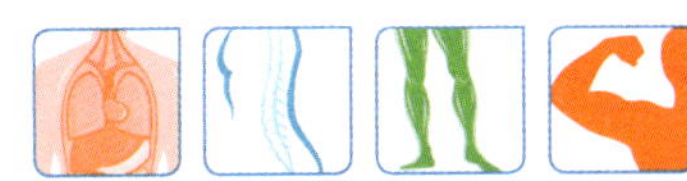

Flow Chart for Bruce Protocol

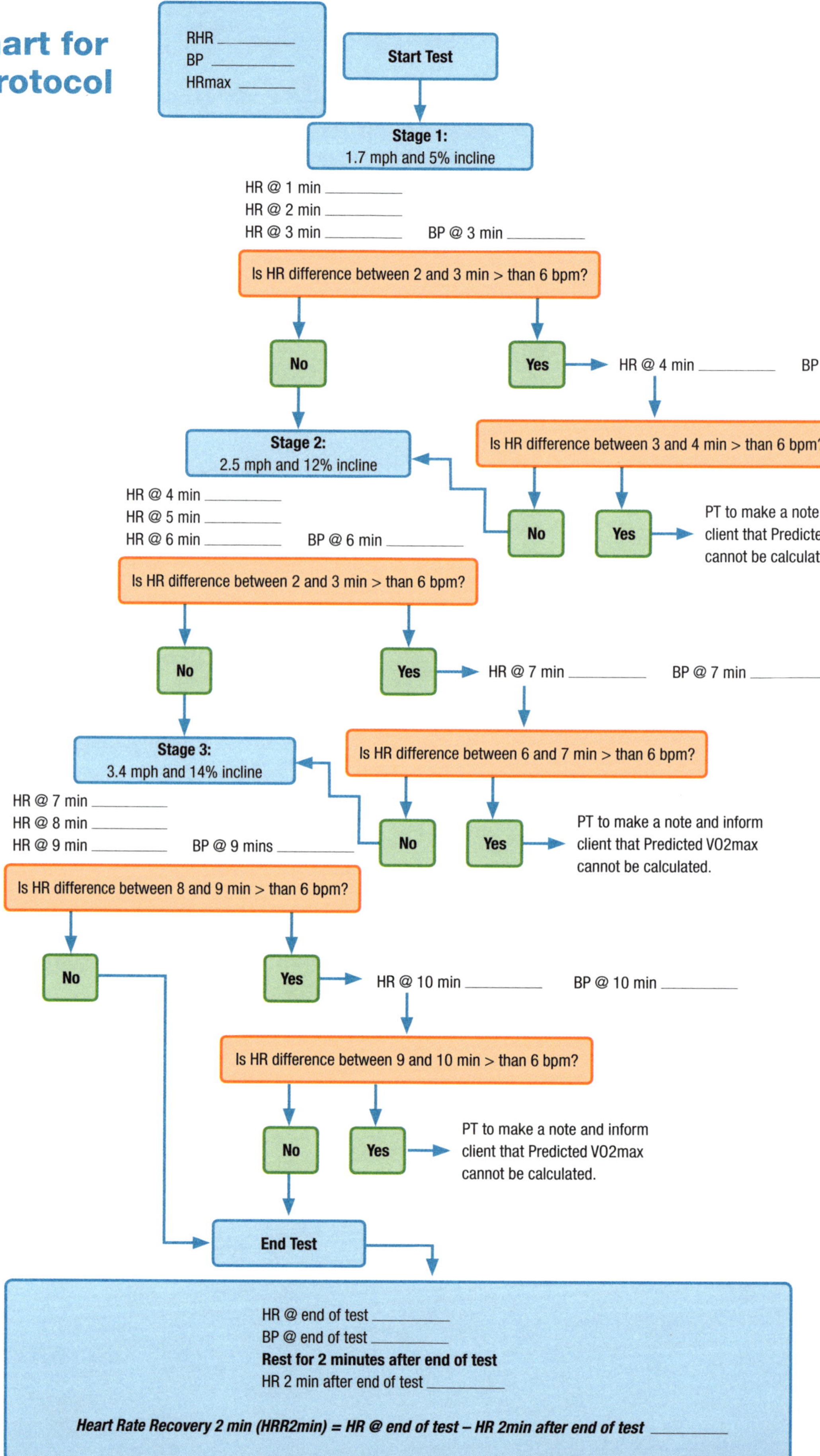

Table 14. Fitness Categories for Heart Rate Recovery After 2 Minutes (HRR2min)

	HEART RATE RECOVERY (HRR2min) (BPM)
Excellent	> 40
Good	36 -39
Average	32 -35
Fair	27 -31
Poor	< 27

Adapted from:
Shetler K, et al. Heart rate recovery: validation and methodologic issues. *J Am Coll Cardiol.* 2001;38(7):1980-1987.
Cole CR, Foody JM, Blackstone EH, Lauer MS. Heart rate recovery after submaximal exercise testing as a predictor of mortality in a cardiovascularly healthy cohort. *Ann Intern Med.* 2000;132(7):552-5.

Table 15. Percentile Values for Maximal Aerobic Power (mL* kg^{-1} * min^{-1})

PERCENTILE	AGE AND SEX									
	20–29		30–39		40–49		50–59		60–69	
	M	F	M	F	M	F	M	F	M	F
90	54.0	46.8	51.7	45.3	49.6	43.1	46.8	38.8	42.7	35.9
80	51.1	43.9	48.3	42.4	46.4	39.6	43.3	36.7	39.6	32.7
70	47.5	41.1	46.0	39.6	43.9	38.1	41.0	34.2	37.4	31.1
60	45.6	39.5	44.1	37.7	42.4	35.9	39.0	32.6	35.6	29.7
50	43.9	37.8	42.4	36.7	40.1	34.5	37.1	31.4	33.8	28.8
40	41.7	36.1	40.7	34.2	38.4	32.8	35.5	29.9	32.3	27.3
30	39.9	34.1	38.7	32.4	36.7	31.1	33.8	28.7	30.8	25.9
20	38.0	32.3	36.7	30.9	34.8	29.4	32.0	26.8	28.7	24.6
10	34.7	29.5	33.8	28.0	32.3	26.6	29.4	24.6	25.6	23.0

Reprinted with permission from: *Physical Fitness Assessments and Norms for Adults and Law Enforcement.* Dallas, TX: The Cooper Institute; 2009. http://www.cooperinstitute.org.

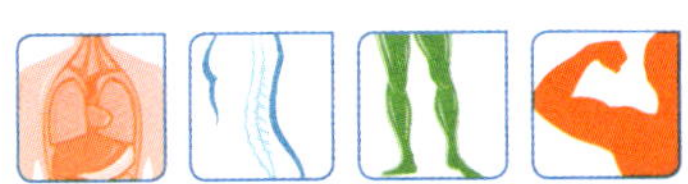

Adult Fitness Examination:

Client Take-Home Form

To the physical therapist:

Fill out the following report after you complete the AFE, and provide a copy to the client.

Adult Fitness Examination

A Physical Therapy Approach

NAME:

DATE:

Following are the results of the Adult Fitness Examination conducted by your physical therapist. Please consult with your physical therapist about any questions you have or actions you want to consider.

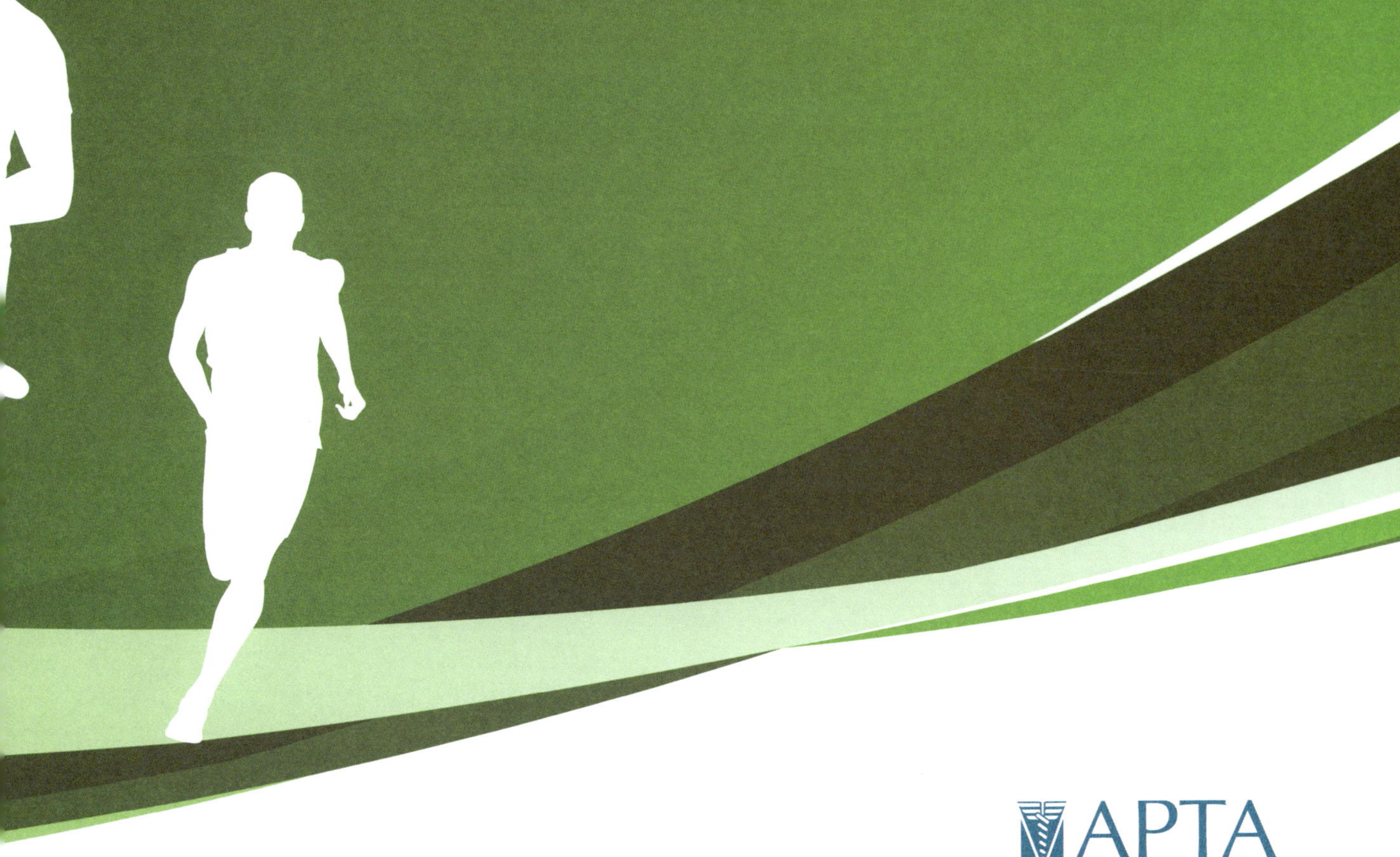

APTA

American Physical Therapy Association

Client's Name: ______________________ **Date of Evaluation:** ____________

Congratulations! You just completed the Adult Fitness Examination. The Adult Fitness Examination, also called the AFE, is a physical therapy approach to define your level of fitness as compared with the general population. This form contains the results of your evaluation.

Cardiovascular/Cardiorespiratory Fitness (Part I)

Normal resting heart rate and blood pressure are an important aspect of cardiovascular/cardiorespiratory fitness. Maintenance of optimal resting heart rate and blood pressure reduce the risk of cardiovascular disease.

RESTING HEART RATE—How hard your heart works without stress

Your Resting Heart Rate is __________ beats per minute

This value is classified as: ○ Bradycardia (heartbeat too slow) ○ Normal ○ Tachycardia (heartbeat too fast)

RESTING BLOOD PRESSURE—How much pressure is in your arteries without stress

Your Resting Blood Pressure is __________/__________ mmHg

This value is classified as:

○ Normal (less than 120/80)
○ Prehypertension (120-139/80-89, potential precursor to high blood pressure)
○ Hypertension, Stage I (140-159/90-99, high blood pressure)
○ Hypertension, Stage II (160+/100+, very high blood pressure)

Comments:

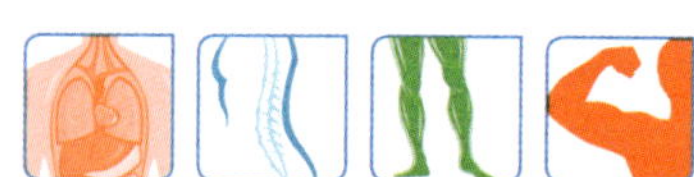

Client's Name: ______________________ **Date of Evaluation:** ______________

Musculoskeletal Alignment and Development

Musculoskeletal alignment and development are important to your overall health in that misalignment can lead to pain and can adversely affect balance, gait, strength, and function. Ideally, proper musculoskeletal alignment is the position in which your joints experience minimal stress, and you require minimal muscle activity to maintain the position.

VISUAL INSPECTION OF POSTURE WITH PLUMB LINE—Alignment and development of your body

Key findings with your posture include: ______________________

____

____

____

Comments:

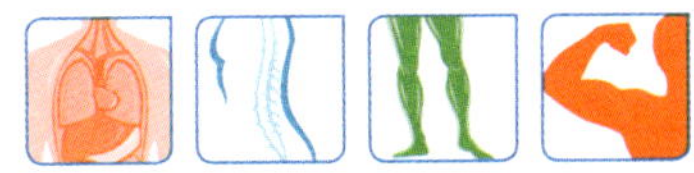

Client's Name: ______________________ **Date of Evaluation:** ______________

Body Composition

Obesity is a major health issue that increases the risk for health conditions such as hypertension, diabetes mellitus, stroke, and coronary artery disease. Body mass index (BMI) combined with waist circumference (WC) are predictors of risk for these conditions.

BODY MASS INDEX—Your weight relative to your height

Your Height is: __________ inches   Your Weight is: __________ pounds

Your Body Mass Index is: __________

This value is: ○ Normal ○ Underweight ○ Overweight ○ Obese ○ Extremely Obese

WAIST CIRCUMFERENCE—The distance around your waist

Your Waist Circumference is: __________ inches

BMI combined with WC indicates disease risk of: ○ Normal ○ Increased ○ High ○ Very High ○ Extremely High

Comments:

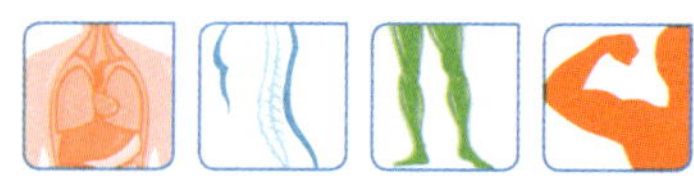

Client's Name: ______________________ **Date of Evaluation:** ______________

Musculoskeletal Fitness: Muscular Flexibility

Musculoskeletal fitness comprises 3 elements: flexibility, strength, and endurance. Flexibility is the ability to move through a range of motion (ROM) without restriction from soft tissue, or capsular or connective tissue elements. Strength is the ability of the muscle to generate maximal force and carry out work against a force. Endurance is the ability of a muscle to perform repeated contractions over time until fatigue. Poor musculoskeletal fitness is associated with possible risk of injury and degenerative joint disease/osteoarthritis.

RANGE OF MOTION (ROM) SCREEN—How flexible your arms and legs are

The flexibility of your arms is:
- ○ Within Normal Limits
- ○ Limitations: ______________________

The flexibility of your legs is:
- ○ Within Normal Limits
- ○ Limitations: ______________________

APLEY'S SCRATCH TEST—Overall shoulder/arm flexibility needed to accomplish everyday tasks such as scratching your back, fastening a bra, or reaching for a wallet in back pocket

With your right arm overhead, left arm behind back, you can/cannot by ________ cm touch fingertips.

With your left arm overhead, right arm behind back, you can/cannot by ________ cm touch fingertips.

YMCA SIT-AND-REACH TEST—How flexible your back and legs are

Your farthest distance reached is: ________ inches

For your age and sex, your percentile ranking is: ________ %

Comments:

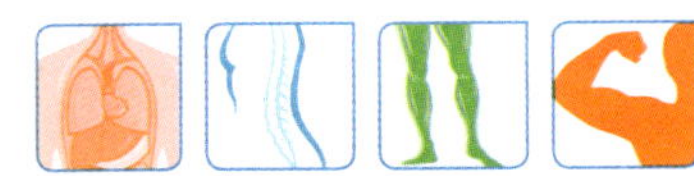

Client's Name: ______________________ **Date of Evaluation:** ______________

Musculoskeletal Fitness: Muscular Strength and Endurance

MANUAL MUSCLE TEST—How strong your arms and legs are

The muscle strength in your arms is: ○ Within Normal Limits
○ Limitations: ______________________

____

The muscle strength in your legs is: ○ Within Normal Limits
○ Limitations: ______________________

____

Comments:

HANDGRIP STRENGTH—How strong your grip is

Your combined right and left handgrip strength is: __________ kg

This result within your age range is: ○ Poor ○ Below Average ○ Average ○ Above Average
○ Limitations: ______________________

____

Comments:

CURL-UP (TRUNK) TEST—Tests the strength and endurance of your abdominal muscles

Number of curl-ups you completed: __________

Your fitness category is: ○ Needs Improvement ○ Fair ○ Good ○ Very Good ○ Excellent

Comments:

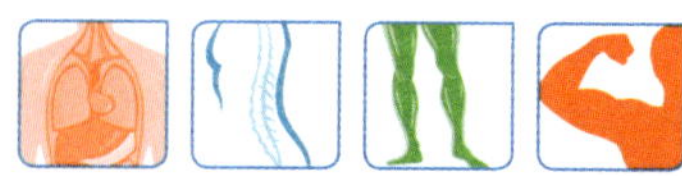

PUSH-UP TEST—Tests the strength and endurance of your upper body and arms

Number of push-ups you completed: ___________

Your fitness category is: ○ Needs Improvement ○ Fair ○ Good ○ Very Good ○ Excellent

Comments:

UNILATERAL STEP-DOWN TEST—Tests the strength and endurance of your lower body and legs

Number of step-downs you completed with your *left* leg: ___________

Your fitness category is: ○ Unable ○ Poor ○ Fair ○ Good ○ Normal

Number of step-downs you completed with your *right* leg: ___________

Your fitness category is: ○ Unable ○ Poor ○ Fair ○ Good ○ Normal

Comments:

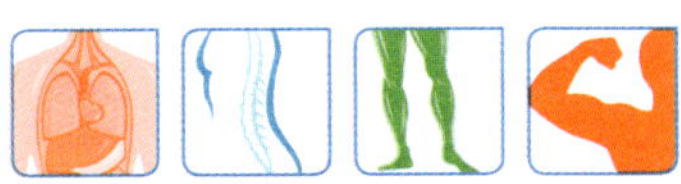

Client's Name: ______________________ **Date of Evaluation:** ______________

Balance

Balance is a major fitness component that is integral to everyday function, as gravity is a constant force. Maintaining balance in the upright position requires complex integration of various systems—the vestibular, somatosensory, and visual systems. Impaired balance contributes to falls, which can lead to impairments and possible disability.

SINGLE LIMB STANCE TEST—Tests your balance on one leg (eyes open and eyes closed)

Your single limb stance balance for your *left* leg, eyes open, is: O Below Norm Value O Above Norm Value
Your single limb stance balance for your *left* leg, eyes closed, is: O Below Norm Value O Above Norm Value

Your single limb stance balance for your *right* leg, eyes open, is: O Below Norm Value O Above Norm Value
Your single limb stance balance for your *right* leg, eyes closed, is: O Below Norm Value O Above Norm Value

O Limitations: ______________________

____

Comments:

UPPER EXTREMITY FUNCTIONAL REACH TEST—Tests your balance when reaching with your upper body (such as reaching for objects on a shelf)

Your average reaching distance is: ________ inches

For your age and sex, you are: O Below Average O Average O Above Average

Comments:

LOWER EXTREMITY FUNCTIONAL REACH TEST—Tests your balance when reaching with your lower body (such as stepping over a hole in the ground)

Your fitness category for the *left* leg is: O Below Average O Average O Above Average

Your fitness category for the *right* leg is: O Below Average O Average O Above Average

Comments:

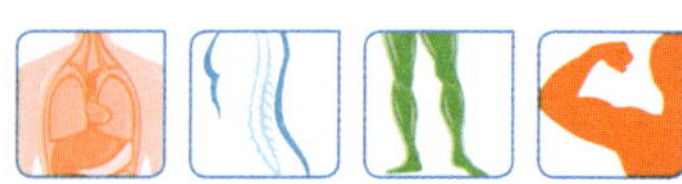

Client's Name: ______________________ **Date of Evaluation:** ______________

Cardiovascular/Cardiorespiratory Fitness (Part II)

Sustained physical activity requires energy for the muscles to function, and that energy comes from oxygen. As the degree of work increases, so does the need to supply oxygen to the functioning muscles. The condition of the cardiovascular/cardiorespiratory systems will dictate the efficacy of energy delivery and, thus, the performance of the task. Poor cardiovascular/respiratory fitness can result in cardiovascular disease, decreased function, and increased morbidity/mortality.

SUBMAXIMAL BRUCE PROTOCOL FOR PREDICTED VO2 MAX AND HEART RATE RECOVERY—

Tests the maximum amount of oxygen your body can consume at the highest exercise intensity you can tolerate (V02max) and how long it takes after exercise for your heart to get back to rest (heart rate recovery)

Your predicted maximal oxygen consumption (VO2max): __________ mL* kg^{-1} * min^{-1}

For your age and sex, your percentile ranking: __________ %

Your heart rate recovery after 2 minutes: __________

Your fitness category is: ○ Poor ○ Fair ○ Average ○ Good ○ Excellent

Comments:

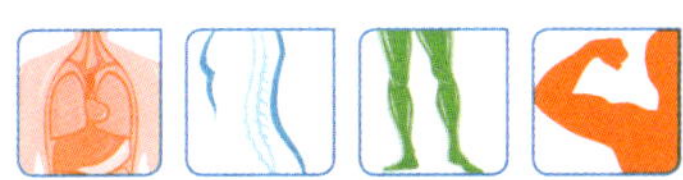

Client's Name: ______________________________ **Date of Evaluation:** ______________

General Comments:

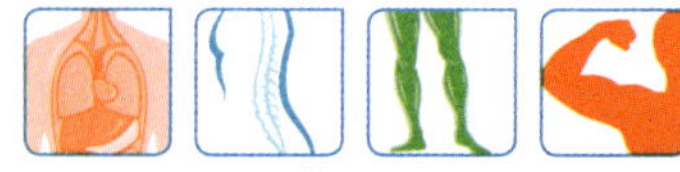